Give Me Strength

Give Me Strength

How I Turned My Back on Restriction, Nurtured the Body I Love, and How You Can Too

ALICE LIVEING

PENGUIN LIFE

AN IMPRINT OF

PENGUIN BOOKS

PENGUIN LIFE

UK | USA | Canada | Ireland | Australia
India | New Zealand | South Africa

Penguin Life is part of the Penguin Random House group of companies
whose addresses can be found at global.penguinrandomhouse.com.

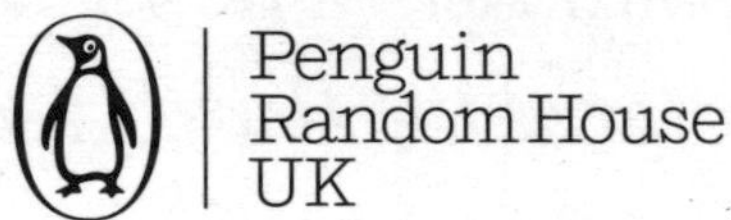

First published 2024
001

Set in 13.5/16pt Garamond MT Std
Typeset by Jouve (UK), Milton Keynes
Printed and bound in Great Britain by Clays Ltd, Elcograf S.p.A.

The authorized representative in the EEA is Penguin Random House Ireland,
Morrison Chambers, 32 Nassau Street, Dublin D02 YH68

A CIP catalogue record for this book is available from the British Library

ISBN: 978–0–241–61896–7

www.greenpenguin.co.uk

Penguin Random House is committed to a sustainable future for our business, our readers and our planet. This book is made from Forest Stewardship Council® certified paper.

For anyone who has thought that being thinner would make them happier, this book is for you

Contents

Prologue

I'm nineteen years old and beyond excited because I've just landed a place at a theatre school in London. It's my first day and I've overcome some pretty hefty obstacles to get here. I feel like I might finally have found a place where I truly belong. I've worked so incredibly hard for it. And – for a brief moment – I really believe I deserve to be here.

Considering some of what I've been through leading up to this point, it's actually a miracle I have the self-esteem to walk into that room at all, let alone the confidence. But I'm doing everything I can to put those difficult memories behind me, and instead look to what I hope will be a bright future. I have taken a risk in being here right now, in following my dreams and turning my back on the 'traditional path' of going to a 'normal' university and then entering corporate life, which maybe my parents expected me to do. And it was all because I hoped to ultimately achieve my lifelong dream of being on the West End stage.

I'd always dreamed of a career as a performer. I spent my childhood learning the lyrics to every musical I saw and spent hours poring over the costumes and the programmes. I was the child who'd put on endless performances at home to anyone and everyone who would watch, often roping in my poor younger brother or cousins, who would serve as bit parts to my starring roles, or simply hold the curtain up as I burst out after the tenth costume change, wearing my mum's old dresses from our bulging dressing-up box. I was the teenager who at every birthday asked for tickets to a West End show and volunteered willingly to be front and centre of every local drama school production. And at some point, I realized that I had to pursue what I knew would make me most happy. I had to pursue my dream of being on stage. The difference between being 'good at dance' at your local stage school and making the leap to performing as a career was huge. I knew that there were no short cuts, but I was determined to get there through sheer hard work and talent. I knew it wouldn't be easy; my dreams of dancing as a prima ballerina had by this stage already been squashed by a dance teacher who said I'd never amount to more than a ballet enthusiast, because of my body shape. But I just refused to believe that I couldn't somehow make it to the point where people were actually paying to see me do the thing I loved most.

I'm standing with my fellow aspiring West End stars, who are dressed like they're ready to burst into a routine from *Chicago* at any minute. There's a huge buzz in the room; the kind you feel on the first day of school when you've got your cool new pencil case and you get to see your friends again after the summer break. Who knows where this is going to take me or who I'm going to become? I try desperately to not be intimidated by the girls in shiny leotards with legs up to their ears.

One of the heads of the college is giving us a pep talk and then we're going to be seen in groups, where we are expected to perform an incredibly fast combination that we've just been taught in five minutes flat. Before dancing, we are each invited into a room for a one-on-one medical.

'Now, Alice,' says the lady running the session. 'If you can just step on to the scales . . .'

And so it begins. *Again.*

Introduction

I should say now that this book is very different to the ones I've written previously. Before I started it, I spent a long time pondering whether it would even be right to revisit some of the things I'm going to talk about in these pages. But on reflection, and with growth, age and therapy, I have realized that there is no better time to address a lot of my journey so far, both on and off-line, and to be open and frank about the realities of it all. About my relationship with my body, the events that warped it, the praise that fed my distorted view, the loneliness that I felt as a result and how, thankfully, I have come out the other side and evolved unrecognizably and irrevocably since then. It has been a difficult journey to live through and perhaps even more difficult to retell, but I hope that in doing so I can share solidarity and hope with other women who deserve to know that they aren't alone. In a world where we're constantly told how we should look, it takes immense strength to resist that narrative. In these pages I want to show you how I found peace with my body and strength both physically and mentally in abundance, and how you can too.

I've been a fitness influencer for almost ten years and

a personal trainer for eight of those. During that time the health and fitness landscape, as well as my approach to my own wellbeing, has changed hugely. Back in 2014 when I founded Clean Eating Alice, it was so normal to see a new diet each week plastered across the media, convincing us that if the previous one didn't work then this one surely would. It was so normal for celebrities to eat themselves bigger, only to lose it all again and come out with a shiny DVD to show us how we could be just like them. The 'no days off', 'no carbs before Marbs', 'no excuses' era was in full flow, and I played my part in it. And now, in 2024, we find ourselves in an incredibly polarized world. At one end of the spectrum you have those who are still heavily entrenched in diet culture and counting calories, exhausting themselves with workouts with the goal of remaining lean. At the other end you have the incredible body positivity movement that has given those in bigger bodies a space to find solidarity and empowerment in a world that is steeped in anti-fat bias. I am absolutely clear that I don't want to take up space in that movement, which is rightly reserved for those women who experience the most stigma. It's also worth noting that the body positivity movement originated from fat, Black and queer activism in response to certain bodies being so rarely visible or held as valuable in discourses and visual media. My intention is to perhaps find something that falls roughly in the middle. While not under a given 'name' as such, I want to speak to women who, like me, want all the joy and benefits that exercise and consistent healthy habits can bring, without obsessing over it.

What I feel is missing, and what I hope to set out in this book, is something that sits between those two extremes. A much kinder, and more realistic way to approach health and fitness that isn't at one end or another. A way that's balanced, enjoyable and – crucially – sustainable. What's difficult about this middle ground is that it's a slightly less sexy sell than the more traditional but quite extreme views of fitness. While the focus isn't shredding yourself day in day out to get rippling abs, it is also not about quitting exercise altogether and just taking it easy 24/7. But – and I speak from experience here – it's an infinitely more realistic and balanced way to engage in positive health behaviours, which will help you on a lifelong journey, rather than just yo-yoing to get yourself ready for and recover from the stress of feeling that you need to be 'beach body ready'. (What a load of rubbish.)

This is why I fully believe that our focus on how we move and feel about our bodies has to improve. Something has to change. Because I don't want to see yet another generation grow up with the same exhausting default of hating their bodies and constantly wanting to make themselves smaller. I want to share the peace I now feel almost every day, with how I exercise and eat, and in the freeing feeling of ridding myself of lifelong shame.

Having spent such a large portion of my twenties totally preoccupied with how flat my stomach felt when

I woke up each morning, it's now a love for my job and my life that gets me out of bed each day. What I've now realized is that without the constant preoccupation of food and exercise swimming around my brain, I have so much capacity to really live – and *enjoy* living. Society has used so many means of keeping women physically and metaphorically small for far too long. (This isn't to say that men aren't also affected by diet culture, they absolutely are, and I hope what I share in these pages will benefit men too.) Whatever your experience up until this point, this book is *your* opportunity to release yourself from the shackles of the control your weight has over you and finally live the life you deserve. It's my personal mission to help you get there.

In the first part of this book, I'm going to share the realities of my journey from the very beginning, looking back at the key moments that led me to where I am now. I reflect on when it seemed to all be going right for me . . . and then how it all went horribly wrong. I'll share how my relationship with fitness began with my love of performing, a passion which set me off on a journey full of problematic relationships and dangerous pitfalls that completely consumed me; as well as how I eventually managed to navigate my way through the undergrowth of toxic diet culture to the place of freedom and balance where I now find myself.

In Part Two, I will set out my four pillars of fitness that have enabled me to find and sustain this balance: Why, What, When, How. Having not only been through my own turbulent journey with fitness, but also having had the privilege of working with thousands of women, in person and online, these pillars are the result of what I have learned about how to approach fitness in a way that prioritizes how it makes you *feel* rather than how it makes you *look*. I have honed and developed these four pillars to show how you can apply them to your own life, no matter where you're at on your journey. There's no pressure, no comparison and absolutely *no* feeling bad about yourself. You can follow it as a sort of plan, or dip in and out and return here whenever you want to reset. That's your choice, and this approach is designed to make you feel good about yourself in every single way.

I feel so passionately about helping people appreciate their body and work out in a way that works for them because I've been there myself: I know exactly how it feels to not be in control or to not know where to start or what to do. I have had a very steep learning curve, and I am genuinely grateful that I've now come out the other side of that tough time in my life. Ultimately, it has made me wiser, braver and helped me find my true purpose, which is helping people achieve body-positive fitness, and I'm so excited to share that with you.

My story

What you'll read over the following pages is an honest account of how I went from a university student simply posting daily updates of my 'healthy' meals online, to becoming one of the most successful fitness influencers at the time. And then how all of that unravelled. I wanted to write this with complete candour, both for my own peace of mind and, more importantly, for you – whether you followed me at the time or not – to get a full picture of what was really happening behind the screen in my life. I think in order to grow and move forward it's important to start from a point of clarity. I realize that some of what I am going to share may be triggering or difficult to read for those of you who followed my apparently rosy journey at the time, and I take responsibility for that. My whole incentive with this book is to try and right those wrongs as best I can and correct the problematic messages that I perpetuated at the time. I feel I've really done the work to get to a place where I can reflect and learn from everything that happened to me, and what I put out into the world as a result. And, in doing so, I want to share those learnings with you too. Saying that, I only encourage you to read on if you feel you are in a strong enough place with your own body right now. Although I think it's important to acknowledge the realities of diet culture so we can speak up against it and find the strength to seek out new narratives, it might not be the right time for you, and that's okay too.

The unfortunate truth is that my journey with my body has followed a similar trajectory to that of many young women, except that it was exacerbated by everything that came with gaining a large online following. My platform really took off in 2016 and between then and the moment that I knew I had to change it, my sole objective was to project the image of someone living their healthiest life. It felt like I was great at something, like people really enjoyed what I was doing; before I knew it, I had this huge following with thousands of people who paid close attention to what I put out there, despite my lack of expertise at the time. While my posts showed a joyously happy, energetic go-getter in matching workout gear, bouncing around from the gym to work to home, there were days when I was so worn out from overexercising and undereating, I would have to build myself up to pose for those pictures before flopping exhausted on to my bed. All my years of performing had paid off as I became an expert in presenting a warped, toned and perfected version of my reality, serene like a swan, when in fact I was madly flailing around under the surface trying to keep the pretence going. Mentally I found myself in a vice, trapped between two realities: on the one hand, I was loving the newfound validation that came from being told I was inspiring, or that I looked amazing, while on the other I knew deep down that my reality was pretty unsustainable and increasingly unenjoyable. Although I did spend most of my days feeling lethargic and low on energy, it wasn't that I couldn't get out of bed each day – I could. But my entire existence was controlled by food and exercise, and so any mental capacity beyond those two things was limited. My social life dwindled, and I reduced most social interactions to controllable circumstances: I either met people for a workout, or at a cafe where I knew the menu well enough to know that I could choose something low calorie that wouldn't affect my overall energy intake for that day. It was all-consuming, and the more I played into the narrative that everything was perfect in my life, the more difficult it became to undo. To put an end to it all. You might be thinking, why didn't you just walk away? I'd be thinking the same. Or you might feel angry at me for pulling the wool over people's eyes. I'd understand that too. So, in the chapters that follow, I have done my best to explain why the cycle was so addictive and how I ended up where I did. And I hope that this isn't where my journey ends either. As I say many times throughout this book, recovery from diet culture and permanently being on a diet takes time; those pesky negative body image thoughts don't disappear overnight. But what I'd like to do is continue this honesty in the hope that women relate to my story, and to do everything in my power to create space for an inclusive world where fitness and body positivity can exist hand in hand.

Fortunately, there came a time when enough was enough, though, and you'll read why later. As awful as it was, I can see now that I needed something extreme to shock me out of the horrendously unhealthy patterns I had come to normalize. Had it not been for that day when I had total clarity, that lightbulb moment of 'shit, something needs to change', I cannot imagine the life I'd be living right now. I certainly don't think I'd have found the joy and love that I have for my job, my relationships and for the little everyday things that I now treasure: my morning breakfast, lazy Sundays on the sofa or sharing a bottle of prosecco with a friend. I am so excited for my future now, but if I hadn't changed my ways, I'm sure that it wouldn't be such a pretty picture. I guess writing this book is the final piece of the puzzle for me in terms of reflecting and learning from where it all went wrong. I've done the work offline, in private, to navigate the tricky pathway that is overcoming eating disorders and the pressures of diet culture and making the many mistakes I did. This now feels like a cathartic end to that journey. A full stop on a period of my life that I'm now able to reflect on objectively and with empathy for myself and those of you reading this who sense similarities between my journey and your own.

If you follow me on social media, you'll be aware that in recent years my attitude, ethos and physique have shifted considerably, and it's been important for me to post about that change fairly regularly. It goes without saying that I am so incredibly grateful that I've had the support of my community throughout this period of my life. When I first began posting online, I used to think that the secret to success was being as small as possible and telling the world how they could diet themselves there too. I'm sure many of you reading this now have had a similar thought process at some point in your lives too, or a moment where you've willed and wished your body to be different. That if only you were smaller, life would be better, people would be kinder, everything would be easier. It's a thought that has probably crossed the minds of most people. And can we blame them? No. There are undoubtedly many benefits to thin privilege that I can attest to. And this idea, this thought process, is a seed planted in our minds from likely as far back as we can remember. If you think back to your earliest memories, I'm sure that among them there are comments or conversations at home, in the playground, on the radio or on TV, which taught you that shrinking yourself was the answer to your problems. And when we do fit the 'ideal', when we do become 'smaller' and join in the never-ending game of body shame and dissatisfaction, we experience the benefits. And so the cycle continues.

I'll be honest, I experienced the 'benefits' of thin privilege myself when I was at my smallest. From the moment my body changed, things started happening for me. I was offered roles in shows where previously I would have been overlooked (at least I thought it was for that reason at the time). I went on to succeed in my career as the first person in my year at theatre school to book a job straight out of college, receiving compliments and adoration. And I was then offered a two-book deal for a six-figure sum by a huge publishing house, despite having very few credentials, all simply because I'd changed my physique. All of this happened when my body changed. But, while I was enjoying all the things that I thought proved how successful I was, I lost sight of how much harm I was doing to my body, not to mention to other people's relationships with food and their bodies. It was only when I eventually woke up to the quite frankly dangerous way I'd been living that I realized just how distracted I'd been by the constant pursuit of trying to remain small. I was living the so-called 'dream' and posting about it, perpetuating this ideal image of health and all the while that just simply wasn't true. That is something I deeply, *deeply* regret.

Acceptance and neutrality

I'm grateful to at last have a body I feel relatively at peace with. I say 'relatively' because, as I said, my main objective is honesty here, and it wouldn't be true to say I'm completely at peace with it. I can have days, weeks, even months where I feel brilliant, and where that niggling voice in my head stays small and silent. But then something will happen and BAM, I'm back in a pit of self-loathing that takes me right back to where I was, and I can spend just as much time crawling out of it and trying my hardest to not slip deeper into the hold of that way of thinking. In the conversations I've had with friends, colleagues, family members and women I have met along the way, I've come to the realization that I don't think I know anyone who is truly 100 per cent happy in their body, and that's okay. And that is why it's so important for me to not paint this rosy picture of 'life after diet culture' as some promised land that you'll be able to get to if only you just loved yourself a little more. I'm a realist, and I want you to know that as much as I want that for you, and for me, it's also far more complex than that. So for now, I settle for the fact that I'm infinitely healthier and happier and everything now works as it should do. And I want you to also reach a similar place. We can't magic away thoughts about our bodies. But we can absolutely change how we respond to those thoughts, and it's this that has helped me most in overcoming body dissatisfaction.

While I am so happy and proud that I'm no longer beholden to the number on the scale or the size of a dress, there's a reason that these things occupy so much unnecessary space in our brains. It's the same reason that we are constantly fed images of the same binary, one-body shape time and time again: it sells! So many powerful industries profit from women, and men, wanting to look different: the beauty, fitness, food and fashion industries – the list goes on. In such a world, we are essentially set up to fail. So it's no wonder so many of us have the same experiences and feelings about our bodies and ourselves. While some might be lucky to avoid the sting of diet culture, for so many of us we end up feeling worse and worse about ourselves, and spending money on anything we can to make ourselves feel more confident and accepted. Which only feeds back into the industry that then continues to harm us and keep us locked in the cycle.

As I say, I don't believe we can just suddenly start

loving every inch of ourselves. I'm too much of a realist to think that way. Instead, I would say a far more useful goal is to strive for body acceptance and neutrality; a completely neutral feeling towards our bodies that means we neither love, nor hate them, we just accept ourselves as we are. It's something that I have tried hard to get to, and I found it a much more possible goal-post. Neutrality feels calm, it feels safe, it feels like your body just becomes less of a priority or focus, and something that takes up less of your headspace. You're not objectifying it, you're not forcing yourself to stand naked in front of a mirror and tell yourself how much you love your body (although by all means do this if you want) but instead, you're just releasing the power that body obsession has over you. That feeling will be fluid; sometimes it's better, sometimes it's worse, but however we feel towards our body doesn't define who we are, or how we show up in the world. And in being neutral we place much less importance on to our bodies, so that we slowly start to think about it less and less.

I come across people all the time, both as clients and online, who've admitted to me that they've hated themselves for twenty, thirty, forty or more years of their life. Imagine, such a huge amount of time spent preoccupied and distracted by an ultimately depressing belief that you're somehow not good enough. For this reason, I do feel it's an impossible task to suddenly just love yourself unreservedly. There is no magic switch that can be flicked that turns off all the negative chatter we constantly say to ourselves as we continue to be fed endless images of people much smaller than ourselves seemingly being the ones that get everything we've ever dreamed of. Instead, by feeling more neutral towards our bodies, and understanding the difference between genuine health and the media's distorted image of health, we can gradually free ourselves from the shackles of diet culture. We can stop questioning every calorie we consume, and every calorie we burn, and win the freedom and headspace to enjoy life to its fullest.

I hope I am proof that you really can learn to accept your body more when you're in a state of balance. Yes, my body has changed, and I'm certainly not as small as I used to be. I accept I will never have a ripped stomach again, nor do I want to, because that's not the way my body is made and it's also not an accurate depiction of my physical health or fitness. But this is the body in which I can truly live my happy, full and rewarding life. It might not be what I imagined my healthiest self would look like, but my goodness is it infinitely healthier than when I spent every single day at the gym and tracked every calorie I ate. This body represents freedom, and I'd take that over being smaller any day.

Finding balance

While it might sound like the solution is to simply stop exercising completely and eat whatever you want, that isn't something I'd necessarily support either. We know that there are some fundamental facts that we must take into account. We know we should all be exercising regularly; it supports our health in so many different ways. Not just our physical strength, but there is evidence of the role that exercise plays in our mental wellbeing, our cognitive function, our energy levels, how well we sleep and even our life expectancy. And we know that eating a balanced and varied diet also supports our brains, our mental wellbeing, our gut and our energy levels. We also know that getting good-quality sleep for 7–9 hours a night is another crucial and well-evidenced piece of our health puzzle. These are all essential elements of health but, crucially, have nothing to do with the way we look. And my days of extreme overexercising and depriving myself of delicious foods, all of which damaged my sleep and caused me endless stress, with the sole aim of winning thousands of likes on Instagram? Needless to say, they're over.

My choice to exercise now comes from a place of self-care and genuine enjoyment. It makes me feel strong, capable and accomplished, which in turn supports my mental health and my overall wellbeing; it creates a part of my identity now, without being the whole of my identity. Previously, I'd walk into a room and want someone to recognize that I was clearly someone who worked out. I don't know why, but I almost wore it as a badge of honour, as if it somehow made me instantly more appealing, and more interesting. Now,

I want people to recognize that I am so much more than someone who works out. I have such a wide variety of interests and passions and friends who both enjoy and don't enjoy working out, and it has become something that I place a lot less value on when it comes to who I see myself as.

It's no longer about how big the gap between my legs is, or whether my arms are as slim as they can be. It's about how I *feel.* And about ensuring that my body stays healthy and strong through all the chapters of my life that are still to come. After years of focusing solely on trying to be 'good enough', by making myself as small as I could, I genuinely feel the best I have ever felt, regardless of the label in the back of my clothes. Happily, that marker of 'success' has now been replaced by much more rewarding, nourishing and fulfilling aspects of life.

The best approach for YOU

What's important to remember as we progress through this book is that I'm not suggesting a one-size-fits-all approach. I'm not dragging out that tired old narrative that if you just follow what I do, your experience and your body will be exactly the same as mine. While we will always be challenged by the deafening dieting racket around us, we need to remember that different bodies respond differently to certain foods and exercise. One person will love CrossFit but hate vegetables, and another person will be the opposite. Genetically too, how we respond to different things matters. That's why this isn't a prescriptive step-by-step solution. Instead, it is about setting out options for you to pick and choose from. I hope you'll also take comfort in the fact that while sometimes it might feel like you're the only person on this journey, I say with kindness and love that you really aren't. I've already helped so many women on this path, and I've learned how many of us struggle in silence with these feelings. You aren't alone, and that is *so* important to remember.

That's why in the second section of this book I've offered a flexible, inclusive, feel-good approach to fitness. I'm not telling you how to look, how much to lift, when to eat or suggesting that you do punishing exercises that will fill you with dread. I'm simply giving you the tools to help you actually enjoy exercise and make it work around you, your preferences and your lifestyle. I'm going to explain everything you need to know about what's important when it comes to moving your body, so that you can make your own decisions as to what feels right for you and where you're at on your journey. And while the methods may vary, I hope the result is that you'll feel genuinely happier and healthier, and perhaps even *finally* free from that exhausting pressure of constantly striving for perfection.

Righting past wrongs

When I first sat down to write this book, I pondered what my mission statement for the overall project should be. Phase one was always to lift the lid and be totally honest about my Clean Eating Alice days, because sharing that is vitally important to me. Rightly or wrongly, I've carried an immense amount of guilt around with me from those days. And while I cannot go back and undo anything that happened, I can reflect on my learnings from a particularly difficult period of my life and share those learnings with you so that those mistakes aren't repeated. But I also wanted to use this time as I looked back to those years to better understand the context that led me and so many others to take such a flawed approach to our health and fitness. And I hoped that by gaining that perspective I could recognize why so many of us find ourselves tied to the constant merry-go-round of diet culture and how I could work to be a positive voice for change in the fitness industry. I knew that while this part of the book was incredibly important, the other part of my mission was to offer a solution to the problem in the best way that I could, in the way that I've had to personally adopt. I have lived and breathed the journey of recovery from those early days to now, and I'm sure there will be many parallels along the way that you might connect to.

I don't claim to have all the answers but when it comes

to fitness, I've pretty much been there, done that and got the T-shirt. I hope that by sharing what I've learned from the many experiences I've had and the errors I've made, I will shine a light on your experience, make you feel seen and help you enjoy moving your body freely again. And perhaps help you to a place where you see your approach to both health and fitness in a whole new way.

The reality is that so many of us have been or are currently on that destructive road of restriction – which is often also (at least in my case) wrapped up in episodes of binge eating and/or excessive exercise and feeling as though you're never quite at peace with your body – and don't know where to turn. Maybe you have experienced an eating disorder, or an unhealthy relationship with exercise, or low self-esteem because of your appearance. Hopefully some of my story will resonate with you and provide much-needed reassurance and advice as to how you can navigate yourself into a better place, both mentally and physically. There is always a way back, and I care passionately about helping you to find it.

One of the more difficult things about having a challenging relationship with our bodies is that it can be incredibly isolating. I get it. More than anything. It can feel as though you're the only one who spends each morning not being able to look at yourself in the mirror. I want my journey to help you feel less alone, feel less ashamed and see that you haven't done anything wrong. Hear me when I say this: none of this is your fault! From the youngest age, we are force-fed the ridiculous diatribe that having a smaller body will make us infinitely happier. Many of us then go on to spend our entire lives trying to be as perfect as possible, navigating huge life shifts like grief, break-ups, pregnancy and menopause, all while trying to convince ourselves that life will be better if we could just fit into the jeans that we wore when we were twenty-one. Imagine being in your eighties and still wishing you were half a stone lighter. That genuinely makes my heart ache.

Letting go of self-loathing

I wish that, just as we see beauty in the diversity of the world around us, we appreciated the differences in our bodies too. For centuries and across cultures, our bodies, particularly women's bodies, have been subjected to scrutiny. This has created an environment in which we constantly feel that the most important and most interesting thing about us is how we look. It can feel as though people's perceptions of us revolve around our outward appearance rather than who we are as people. As women, we have had our bodies policed by men, and our beauty standards created by those in positions of power who want us to buy things from them. We've been taught to compete with other women, and we've been told what's 'hot' and what's 'not' by every tabloid magazine going. Rather than being angry at the magazine plastering unkind photos of some celebrity whose body shape may have changed on the cover, we absorb the subtle messaging that to gain weight is to fail. And so, consciously or subconsciously, that sense of shame can creep in any time you fluctuate in shape. This is particularly pertinent when paired with the shaming of women who choose to do things differently and carve their own narrative. Often the women who don't conform to the beauty 'blueprint' suffer backlash from mainstream media who will do their best to ridicule and shame them. Lizzo springs to mind here, although there are of course others.

It's interesting to cast your mind back and see if you can remember a time when you weren't aware of the size or shape of your body. Was there a time when you didn't wake up every morning and look in the mirror to evaluate if you look bigger or smaller than the day before? Do you have days where you choose something from your wardrobe with confidence, knowing it will fit and you will feel good? And others where you agonize over what you can 'get away with' that day? (Generally, anything oversized that doesn't make you feel self-conscious or uncomfortable. Am I right?)

Of course, there are many other factors at play when it comes to the way we perceive and treat our bodies, some of which I talk about in my own story, but there is no denying that the media is largely responsible for how we feel about our bodies. I distinctly remember as a teenager seeing magazines that would gleefully photograph celebrities in slightly bigger bodies and caption them 'she's let herself go', or 'shows off her curves'. And let's not forget the notorious 'best' and 'worst' dressed lists. We found ourselves literally being told how to conform to the narrowest of beauty standards, or else we'd be deemed unattractive, uncool or out of touch. I often hear people older than me saying how grateful they are to have grown up before the likes of Instagram and TikTok existed. But the reality is that for as long as advertising and mainstream media have been around, there has been an unrealistic representation of women, and men, impressed upon us, creating a disconnect between our reality and what we feel like we *should* look like.

'Ideal' women

Idealized images of women are nothing new. Google adverts from the 1950s and you'll find photos of stereotypically gorgeous women dreaming about getting vacuum cleaners for Christmas. Always in slim bodies, always perfectly pristine with their coiffed hair, blemish-free skin and pearly white teeth. The narrative is clear: this is what you should aspire to look like. Here is your beauty ideal. On the one hand, I'm grateful that at least we've moved on from the days where every message was gendered and women were expected to stay at home and raise children (while looking perfect, of course).

And yet, as the decades have passed, the message has been neatly packaged up in many different formulas but remains almost entirely the same. Films and TV shows today are still, for the most part, filled with women who look like they've walked out of the pages of a fashion magazine. Women who find themselves in bigger bodies are the 'funny' ones, or the girl who wears glasses is the 'clever' one. And there's the timeless story of 'woman changes her appearance and suddenly falls in love'. *Friends* was one of my favourite shows as a child, but now I'm shocked to think back to the storyline about Monica's weight, how 'fat' and unattractive she used to be, compared to how gorgeous she became. Her weight was a recurring joke throughout the show, and I laughed along at the time, but on reflection, I realize just how confronting this casual take must have been for anyone existing in a slightly bigger body. It is just one prime example of how insidious the messaging is around how making ourselves smaller makes us infinitely more attractive and desirable.

It begs the question: without the media projecting these narratives, would we feel the same pressure to 'fix' ourselves to fit into an ever-shifting ideal of what we should look like? When I was growing up, there were very few celebrities bar Dawn French who didn't fit the 'ideal' body shape. And even then, her weight was always front and centre of her comedy and made fun of. There are countless stories of models, who already had incredibly small bodies, being asked to diet further to fit impossibly tiny high-fashion sample sizes. If that doesn't prove women can't win, what does? If even a supermodel can be told that they're not quite small enough, what message does that send to the rest of us? And this issue isn't solely reserved for women. While I think women do bear the brunt of the pressure from the world around them, neither have men escaped the narrative that they should embody a certain look to be more desirable and to fit the 'ideal' physique. Men have long been told that, unlike women, being muscular is key to their 'success'. Again, we only need to look to the narrow representation of men in adverts, on social media and in films to realize that there is also a very unattainable muscular body image that they are bombarded with. Who gets to say what kind of body is okay and what isn't? Who says people can't have lumps and bumps and breakouts, and hair that has frizzy, out-of-control days? Whatever your gender, it goes without saying that the constant feelings of inadequacy are draining.

Where does this come from?

The hardest thing about it all is that we aren't all born hating the way we look. In the next chapter, I share some of my fondest memories of eating, playing, moving and living freely and without any feeling of judgement from the outside world or from within me. It may have been a long time ago, but all of us can likely remember a time when we were completely at ease with our bodies. A freeing feeling of not caring about taking your clothes off at the end of the day, and not worrying about how you looked before every holiday. When you ate what you wanted without checking the calorie content or worrying about needing to exercise to 'burn off' the food you'd consumed the day before. Maybe you are already in that happy place and you never worry about those things, and that's brilliant. But the likelihood is, because of the environment in which we exist and the culture we're all influenced by, that niggling feeling is often there at the back of your mind.

When I began writing this book, I realized that across the many conversations I've had with women over the years, whether with my clients, friends or strangers I've interacted with, the majority of us *will* have experienced a period in our lives when we didn't fear food. A time when fullness and hunger weren't shameful or things to be suppressed, or when you got out of breath from running around just for the fun of it. Perhaps for you, that means thinking way back to being a small child; for many of us, that's the last time we remember eating or moving without the ever-deafening internal chatter getting in the way. But I didn't want to speak purely subjectively about my own experiences, I wanted to get a better understanding of what the research says about our relationships with our bodies, food and fitness. Sadly, it was a pretty depressing task. One study I read found that 34 per cent of five-year-old girls engaged in deliberate dietary restraint at least 'sometimes'. The same study found that 40 per cent of girls aged between five and nine wish they were thinner. This is clear evidence that disordered behaviour begins achingly young for so many of us. These statistics are awful to read, but what's clear is that we are not born with this inner turmoil around food, or with anxiety about our body shape. It's something the environment in which we grow up teaches us. We live in an objectifying world that educates us from birth that we *are* our bodies, and therefore our appearance defines our worth. It's no wonder so many of us find ourselves on a near-lifelong cycle of shame and dieting.

It is heartbreaking that this preoccupation with self-image starts from such a young age, a time when we should be free of worries and self-doubt. In another study, a group of researchers at Williams College in the US explored children's relationships to body image and anti-fat bias. Researchers told stories to children aged three to five, in which one child was mean to another child. Afterwards, the researchers showed the kids pictures of other children who ranged from thin to chubby, and they were asked which child was the mean one. The children in the study assumed it was the chubby child. When asked which child they would most like to play with themselves, they were less likely to want to play with the chubby child, demonstrating how we are conditioned to develop an anti-fat bias from a very young age.

This unconscious bias that we absorb from the

language and attitudes around us throughout our lives can then dictate our perception of what is acceptable and what isn't. Unsurprisingly, data also shows that women experience the consequences of this to a much greater degree than men. For example, one study published in the *International Journal of Eating Disorders* in 2015 found that women were sixteen times more likely to experience weight-based discrimination in a workplace setting than men. This shows clearly that while men aren't immune from shame and body image issues, larger male bodies are far more socially acceptable than larger female bodies.

A new way

I'd like to think that things *are* changing. There is undoubtedly more diversity across the adverts that I see today compared to when I was a teenager, for example. And we are fortunate to now have incredible examples of women bucking the trend of apparently needing to be 'thin' to be successful; think of Lizzo, Alison Hammond, Melissa McCarthy, Megan Jayne Crabbe and Ashley Graham, as well as countless influencers online (Remi Bader is my favourite). But the reality is that things aren't changing quickly enough.

We definitely don't need another interpretation of how we *should* look. We just need to be able to freely exist in varying shapes and sizes, as nature intended.

We need so many more positive role models than we have currently because the reality is that we cannot be what we cannot see. It will always be difficult to accept ourselves when we don't see similar people reflected in magazines, on TV, online and in advertising. It should be the norm that we see a full range of body types modelling clothes, as well as in the fitness industry.

What I did was follow the supposed formula for success down to a tee. I shrank myself down in the hope of finding that magical pot of gold at the end of the fat-loss rainbow . . . before I realized that it doesn't exist. If anything, I was even more disappointed and miserable than before, but with a new-found and exhausting preoccupation with food and exercise.

I don't have everything nailed now, and I don't want this book to seem to come across as a 'just be like me, it's so easy' kind of shtick. I know it isn't that easy. And I still have days that I find challenging, when that little voice in my head tries to convince me I'd be happier smaller. But, for the most part, I feel ready and able to talk about my experience and how I've worked to have far, far more good days than bad. It is important for me to be as honest as I can possibly be in this book, and some of it may make for difficult reading. It all comes from a good place and I want it to be helpful and a catalyst for change. But, as a trigger warning, some of the content is sensitive. If you feel like you may be challenged by references to eating disorders and excessive exercise, I want to give you a heads-up now, so you can choose whether you want to continue. If you recognize these behaviours in yourself now or at any point throughout the book and think there is a possibility of it being an eating disorder, please do acknowledge it and seek help. The team at eating disorder charity Beat are wonderful – with their help I have included a list of resources at the end of the book.

I also want to say that in writing this book, I don't want my help to simply end here. I have recognized in myself the power of sharing my story with others and of finding experiences and similarities in others' journeys. With that in mind, I want to extend the opportunity to you to reach out to me online at any time if you're struggling. You're not alone, and this stuff can be complex to work through, so please do feel free to lean on me if you need to.

Love always,
Alice x

PART ONE

Me

1. Where it all started

I grew up in Buckinghamshire in a small town called Gerrards Cross. I lived in a house with my loving parents and my older sister and younger brother. Life was relatively calm and full of fun and, as with most children, my days, while full of school and activities, were punctuated by three mealtimes. Food was delicious and abundant in our house and forms a big part of a lot of my earliest memories. My mum is Jewish and her upbringing taught her so much about the role of food within the family. Every Friday in her household, and instilled in us from a young age, was the gathering for Shabbat. Her mum (my grandmother) would pour love and care into making a meal for sometimes twenty plus people every Friday without fail, and it was often said that food was the beating heart of the family. My mum has always been an excellent cook – her mother taught her to cook but also showed her the effect good food could have on bringing a family together – and she'd spend hours preparing wholesome home-cooked meals such as fish pie and spaghetti Bolognese that we'd all enjoy as a family. I vividly remember running out of the school gates at home time and immediately asking my mum what was for dinner. It wasn't because I was fussy, or because I cared about what was in the meal. Quite the opposite, it was because I knew that whatever was waiting for me at home was going to be delicious, and I was already looking forward to eating it. This was an innocent time when the only thoughts I had about food bounced between being hungry and excited to eat, or joyfully eating whatever was in front of me. There was no mental maths of how many calories might be in whatever I was being served, or whether it contained too many carbohydrates. I was simply savouring food in a 'normal' and natural way.

There are particular memories that I really cherish from that time. My mum would make the most incredible desserts, my favourite being an Eton mess, which she'd create with smashed meringues, squirty cream and berries. I'd devour every sweet, sticky mouthful before immediately going back for seconds. The language around food at home never made me feel this was anything but ordinary and it meant that I honoured my body's signals telling me when I was hungry and when I was full. To lots of you this might sound like I'm stating the obvious, but this level of intuitiveness was a luxury that I was completely unaware of at the time. It meant that I didn't spend hours thinking about food, or ruminating about what I wanted to eat versus what I should eat. I ate what I was given, and I rarely snacked between meals as I was eating plentiful portions that left me satisfied.

I feel lucky that for the most part I was shielded from any body issues until around the age of eleven or twelve, but I can vividly remember the period when everything changed. At my new all-girls secondary school, eating was discussed a *lot*. Calories and fat content – things I'd never considered before – were a constant part of everyday conversations and made me much more aware of what I put in my mouth. The way other girls talked to each other and how food was discussed made it clear that what we ate was important, and if you wanted to be slim, avoiding certain foods was even more important. It's incredible to think how we must have absorbed and accepted those beliefs from our family homes, magazines or TV without question and then parroted them back to each other as gospel. Rather than being able to enjoy food together, mealtimes became an opportunity for comparison. I still remember the feeling of picking up a dessert bowl and then swiftly placing it back down. Not because I didn't want dessert, but because I didn't want any of my friends to see me eating it. It was as if every mealtime became a moment of pressure where making the 'right' choices meant forgoing the foods you really wanted. And so the pressure to be thinner began to impact more and more of my beliefs and my sense of self.

Becoming a teenager meant that along with raging hormones came a lot of physical changes within my body, many of which I didn't like. My recollection was that, unlike my friends, my boobs seemed to develop pretty quickly, and they were something that I was instantly embarrassed about. I distinctly remember a conversation with one of my friends at the time who informed me that 'the bigger your boobs, the fatter you were, because boobs were made out of fat'. This comment brought about instant shame and was the start of me feeling as if I needed to hide my body in baggier clothes to cover the fact that I felt bigger than the other girls in my friendship group.

As I became more conscious of my changing body, it wasn't just that I felt the need to hide it, I also found myself increasingly questioning the food I ate and the exercise I was doing. At thirteen years old, you can imagine the impact that then had on my energy and ability to learn. I was becoming more easily distracted in classes and drifting off into deep daydreams that often felt like I was asleep with my eyes open. Even now I question whether I might have done 'better' at school had I not been so preoccupied with this obsession with being smaller, and whether I would have enjoyed lessons more if I'd had a proper amount of energy in me to actually take on the information I was being taught.

Looking back it's clear that we had no filter and very little understanding of the impact our words and behaviours had on each other. In hindsight, it is really upsetting that we were judging each other's figures as young as thirteen, but at the time it seemed completely normal to comment on girls with slightly bigger bodies in a negative way. I look back now and cringe at the harmful rhetoric that my friends and I perpetuated, but I share this now to show how normalized it was to judge anyone who differed even slightly from the 'norm'.

I remember dabbling with what I now know to be

restrictive eating around the age of fourteen. I didn't know that it had a name at the time, it just meant I was more aware of what I was eating and consciously chose to eat less. The canteen where we ate lunch became strangely intimidating and I quickly sensed how those who finished their whole plate or ordered foods like pizza or chips were judged. We were all anxious to conform, to do the 'right' thing and with these behaviours came a sense of moral superiority, as if somehow abstaining from foods that I really wanted to eat meant that I was better than those who didn't. I remember feeling hungry at times and yearning for the desserts and snacks on offer at school, but I soon learned that hunger was purely a by-product of achieving a smaller body, which was ultimately far more important. It was a time when having some crazily thin model or celebrity as your background was supposed to be 'motivation' and your MySpace was littered with quotes such as 'sweat is just your fat crying' and 'nothing tastes as good as skinny feels'. We were children born in the nineties and growing up in the noughties, with the hangover of the power of thinness during those years still very much present. Thin was still in, and we were living proof of the reality of that movement and the impact it had on young girls like me.

Around this time, while I was in Year 9 it was very clear that I'd subscribed to what I believed was a 'healthy' way of eating. Food now occupied a great deal of my headspace and it seeped into my home life as well. Instead of skipping out of school excited for my mum's dinners, I now worried about how much pasta my mum was serving me, and asked if she could sub out potatoes for vegetables for me in other dishes. Without realizing, I had sleepwalked into a controlled relationship with food. Everything had shifted and I had lost the childhood innocence of simply enjoying what I was eating.

Breaking the cycle

It was around this time, as my preoccupation with food grew, that I began to notice my mum's relationship with food. I guess up until this point I hadn't paid much attention to how other people chose to eat, but suddenly I was picking up on behaviours that I clearly recognized in myself. I remember becoming conscious of Mum's constant dieting. As soon as I entered the world of dieting and restriction, I could see in my mum the exact same behaviours that I was starting myself. In fact, I have very little memory of when she *wasn't* on a diet, which makes me desperately sad. Since opening up about my own journey over the last few years, we've talked a lot about how difficult that time was for her. She had struggles with her own body image throughout my childhood, which led to disordered eating issues, but she kept my sister and I sheltered from them for as long as she could. Knowing this now, she must have worked incredibly hard to avoid showing us the reality of her relationship with food. Although I eventually spotted certain behaviours that mirrored my own, she had always encouraged us to eat a full and varied diet. It was only as my own relationship with food and my body started to become more complicated that it became clear that, to some extent, I was simply copying what my mum was doing. This also seeped into how we spoke about bodies at home and when we were out. I started to notice that my mum could be incredibly disparaging about those who occupied bigger bodies, and she'd pass comment on people who might have gained weight. We'd be out and about together, perhaps sat having a tea and she'd say, 'Gosh look at how big that woman is,' or 'Blimey, can you believe she's wearing that?' Because of her own internalized fat-phobia, I absorbed a lot of this messaging and ended up thinking the same way she did whenever I saw someone in a bigger body or someone who had put on weight, like it was this terrible thing, which of course slotted in perfectly with what I was learning from my peers at school. What my mum was subconsciously teaching me is what she was taught too. Fat is bad, and those who occupy bigger bodies are fair game to be talked about in a negative way. And, of course, talking about those in bigger bodies naturally made us feel better about ourselves.

With my compassionate hat on, I now totally understand it. She was sadly only repeating and regurgitating the stuff she'd been taught by her own mother. I mean, my poor mum was put on WeightWatchers aged twelve, as if that was a totally normal thing to do. No wonder she felt the pressure to be thin, and to criticize those who weren't. It wasn't just her relationship with food that suffered either. I saw my mum restrict and punish herself with exercise constantly. She went running even though she hated it, and spent a lot of money on expensive personal trainers. Why? Because she had spent her formative years learning how crucial it was to be slim as a woman, and she just wanted to be accepted. As do we all. And so, like her, my relationship with exercise, beyond doing compulsory PE lessons at school, was that you exercised when you wanted to lose weight, and that was it. It was a way to punish yourself should you stray from the strict dieting rules you tried to stick to. You worked out, which at the time meant running on a treadmill until you hit a certain calorie target, as well as nightly sit-ups before bed after a big meal the night before; you worked out more before a holiday and you worked out all the time when your goal was to shrink yourself. Enjoyment didn't even come into the equation. There was one time that I went with my mum to one of her personal training sessions, and there was another lady there who dashed out to be sick mid-workout because she hadn't yet eaten that day – it was 2pm. But this was almost seen as the ultimate commitment. I actually think about that moment a lot and how much of an impression it made on me, seeing this woman be so ill but then come right back in and carry on working out as if nothing had happened. Even at the time I realized that that was surely an excessive commitment to the cause of being 'in shape'. My impression until then had been that if you were sick, you were ill and needed to rest. But seeing this woman and how determined she was to get back into the gym despite clearly being unwell skewed my entire understanding of what I believed to be true. This experience imbedded the dangerous idea in me that thinness was more important than acknowledging illness. Her long, blonde flowing hair and lean limbs told me that this is what true commitment looks like. Knowing what I know now about how impressionable we are as young people, and how we often directly copy or mimic what our parents do, it's clear that on some level these messages infiltrated my idea of what health and fitness looked like. And so the vicious cycle continued with me.

Now, this is by no means a blame game; I'm not in any way holding my mother or my grandmother or anyone else in my life responsible for the situation I found myself in. In fact, I think it's crucial to understand that nobody is to blame, and yet everybody is to blame at the same time. It's not one person, it's all of us, repeating these impossible standards, displaying them in full view for the next generation of teenagers, with nobody questioning why. Why do we need to be thin? Why are we taught that exercise is only there to keep us small? Why do we have to question and scrutinize everything we eat? Instead, we accept and repeat. It's impossible to see it when you're in the thick of it, but I'm so happy that I now, finally, understand the context of how my journey with diet culture began, and how it led me down the path it did. I have since had so many conversations with my mum about this time, and how difficult it was for her. If I am ever lucky enough to have a family of my own, I am determined to do everything in my power to break the cycle.

The male gaze

Our teenage years are a time when we're desperate to just fit in and be liked; we crave a sense of validation like never before, whether that be from friends and peers, or from the opposite sex who we are just starting to interact with. My school was single-sex from Years 7 to 11 but there was an equivalent all-boys school to my all-girls school, and my classmates and I regularly socialized with the boys there. So in Years 8 and 9, just as I was becoming hyperaware of my body, what I was eating and how to fit in with my friends, I was also starting to deeply crave validation from boys. I became more conscious of my body when I started wondering how boys would feel about it. I so wanted to be pretty and the girl that people fancied. I remember how the boys would constantly assess who had a 'good body' – they almost always meant girls who occupied smaller bodies than I did. It was like a gut-punch hearing them list girls smaller than me and I remember lying awake some nights literally wishing and willing myself thinner, as if that would be the ticket to being likeable. Reflecting on this period in my life, it's interesting to me that what started as low-level feelings of unhappiness in myself and my physique were totally exacerbated by thoughts of how other people would feel about me rather than how I felt about myself. That feeling of not being desired reinforced the idea that I wasn't thin enough; that how thin I was linked both to how successful and how attractive I was. I seemed to care more about how other people saw me than how I saw myself. I can't speak for all my peers, but I don't think this feeling of inadequacy was out of the ordinary. Our size was our identity; it determined how worthy we were to others, but also to ourselves.

This pressure to be as small as possible loomed over me throughout school but there were definitely trigger points when that fear of judgement felt even more intense. The need to look a certain way could overtake any other worries I had at the time. For example, in the weeks running up to sports days, rather than practising the event (usually the relay) that I was participating in so that I didn't come last, I'd be more worried about restricting my food because I had to wear my sports kit in front of boys (who we shared our sports day with). Similarly, whenever there was a party or event out of school hours when we could wear our own clothes, how I looked was of the utmost importance. I would have a hyper focus on the foods I was eating, which had nothing to do with *health* and everything to do with how much weight I could lose. My interpretation of nutrition at the time meant that I didn't have any understanding of the importance of fruits and vegetables, or protein, for example. Instead, I thought the Special K diet was the best way to lose weight (didn't we all fall for this one at some point)? This meant that there were many days where I took my 'lunch' to school, stuffed into my blazer pocket, consisting of a crunched-up bag of Special K in a ziplock bag. No milk. No flavour. It was essentially like chewing slightly sweetened cardboard for lunch. God it was miserable, and for what? It wasn't like anyone actually paid me a compliment or showed any greater interest in me than before.

Our school years are formative in so many ways, especially when it comes to our first romantic relationships. Like all my friends at the time, I did everything in my power to try and fit the shape and size that boys seemed to like, to get their attention and feel worthy. Some of my friends found themselves in happy relationships that lasted weeks, even months, usually ending in tears before moving on to the next, but my experience was quite different and ended up changing me as a person for ever. When I look back at this period of my life, it almost feels unreal. The woman I am today is so vastly different from the girl I was, and I am still almost in disbelief that these events happened to me. I feel so far from that person and that place now. It's funny how whole chunks of our lives can become a total blur as we whirlwind through tumultuous and traumatic life experiences. Thankfully, with the help of an incredible therapist, I've managed to piece together this part of my life and get to a point where I now feel very comfortable talking about it.

*

As a teenager living in a small town with my family, I desperately wanted to be more independent. There wasn't a huge amount to do in Gerrards Cross. Our best offerings of entertainment were the local cinema and a roller disco that took place every Friday evening at the local leisure centre. As I got older, I wanted nothing more than to be able to go out on my own and explore the big wide world. I remember having numerous shouting matches with my mum, as teenagers do, trying to convince her to let me go out and do things like going to the nearest shopping centre on my own. Having an older sister meant I saw all the exciting things the world had to offer through her; I was so envious of her and craved adulthood from a young age. Whenever I could, I was out of the house doing all the things I thought a teenager should be doing: hanging around the shops, going to parties, staying out as late as possible. While it makes me cringe now, I remember the freedom of being out and about with my friends, sat on the local common thinking I was so cool. It was on one such occasion – when I'd lied to my mum and pretended I was going for an innocent sleepover at a friend's house, but was in fact going to a house party – that I met my ex.

I was sixteen years old, just finishing my GCSEs, and desperately wanting a boyfriend who would make me feel like the adult I wanted to be. My experience of meeting boys outside of school was pretty non-existent, or at least meeting any that I liked, and my all-girls school clearly provided no options, so when I met him that night for the first time, he seemed to be everything I wanted. He drove a car, which meant independence. He was older than me, which meant adulthood felt that much closer. He smoked, which I thought was cool. It sounds like such a cliché that those were the things that drew me to him, but I was young and desperate for a taste of real life, so I can empathize with that younger version of me and everything she thought she wanted. We all make dating mistakes, especially as teenagers, right?

From day one, we started seeing each other regularly and became 'exclusive' after only a matter of weeks. Unlike many teenage relationships, where things progress gradually as you get to know each other, ours went from 0 to 100 in a matter of days. One week we were strangers, the next we were spending absolutely every free moment together. Even if we had spent all weekend together, when we said goodbye, he'd be sending me messages asking to see me again. And it wasn't just that we spent all our time together. From early on, he showered me with affection, buying me gifts I didn't ask for and making me feel special, which I think most sixteen-year-olds would be flattered by. I enjoyed the thrill of it to begin with, driving around together in his car, even if it was just to the shopping centre or to get a McDonald's and sit in the car park. At the start, he did make me feel special, and that disarmed a lot of my body worries. I began to relax around food more and enjoyed going out for nice meals or getting a takeaway together, which was something I previously would have felt guilty about. I finally had the freedom I had craved away from my family and school, but deep down I knew there was something not quite right. I guess even from the start of the relationship I knew that he didn't set my world alight, and by that I mean he wasn't someone I'd thought I'd end up with. He smoked and had dropped out of education, two things that were a little out of my comfort zone, but he made me feel desired, he made me feel special, and he ticked enough of the boxes that I thought needed ticking, and that seemed enough of a reason to continue the relationship.

It felt like a teenage infatuation from a movie; we had just met and then suddenly we were inseparable. Looking back on it with the perspective I have now, it seems crazy that I flipped my life upside down for this person overnight, but it was my first love. Of course, my family weren't happy about me disappearing for hours, even days at a time, but I was all-consumed by what I thought was an adult relationship. My friends had done it, I'd seen it on TV, and now it was my turn. In my naive eyes, he just seemed to care about me a lot, and wanting to spend all his time with me was incredibly flattering. Remember that at this point in my life my confidence was pretty low and my need for external validation was pretty high. My lack of self-confidence meant that whenever someone showed me love and attention, I lapped it up unquestioningly. The relationship progressed from barely knowing each other to now spending every free moment outside of school with him, and for a while, everything seemed good. That is, until it wasn't.

The first time he hit me, I remember being stunned to complete silence. We'd been in the car travelling home from a football match. It was a chilly winter day and I'd spent three hours of my weekend wrapped up on the sidelines cheering him on as he played for a local team. As we drove to the game, nothing was untoward. We'd had breakfast together and chatted happily on the journey to the football group. But once the game was over, something changed. He had this look in his eyes that I'd never seen before, but I couldn't understand why. His team hadn't lost. He hadn't had any rough altercations from what I could see. And yet something was definitely wrong. As he loaded his kit into the car, he slammed the car boot, which startled me. I didn't know how to respond so I just acted as though everything was normal, desperate to try and transport us back to the happy bubble that we'd been in just a few hours ago. But as the conversation progressed it turned out that he'd taken issue with me talking to one of his friends on the sidelines. This was baffling to me. His friend? The one who chatted to me for just a few minutes about the game and how freezing we were? I couldn't get my head around it, so I asked what on earth he'd thought I'd said or done. And then . . .

The sting of the slap paralysed me in shock; I didn't cry or scream. As his blind rage turned to profuse apologies, I remember that shock turning to confusion. The person who just a few hours ago was talking about us booking our first holiday, the person who had become my world, who was supposed to care about me had just attacked me for no reason. There was no script for what to say next and I just wanted things to go back to the way they were so then *I* started to apologize for not accepting his apologies quickly enough. As my apologies turned to tears, I sobbed in total helplessness. He hugged me and after we'd both said 'sorry' and 'I love you' a few more times he started the car to drive home. As I stared out of the window, tears still streaming down my face, I started to replay the events of that day over and over. Was I to blame? Had I been a bit flirty with his friend? Deep down I think I knew I hadn't done anything wrong, but I started to doubt myself.

Knowing what I know now, this is a classic example of how gaslighting works. This form of emotional abuse can be incredibly hard to spot and even harder to call out. For those of you who have heard of it but perhaps don't truly understand what gaslighting is, I'd like to take a moment to explain. Gaslighting is a form of emotional abuse that causes a victim to question their own feelings, instincts and sanity. As a result, the abusive partner has a lot of power and control over them. Once an abusive partner has broken down the victim's ability to trust their own perceptions, the victim is more likely to stay in the abusive relationship. So, as you can see, for me and millions of other women across the world, being constantly undermined and coerced means that you start to question everything you do. And, in cases like mine, you start to believe that you are to blame.

That moment in the freezing cold car park was just the

beginning of the abuse, but it was the gaslighting that kept me in that relationship. It was the gaslighting that kept me constantly questioning whether it was my fault, whether I was provoking his outbursts and bad tempers, his jealousy and attacks that came out of the blue.

This pattern of behaviour – abuse, apology, regret, showering me with love, followed by abuse, apology, regret and again, showering me with love – sadly worsened and became more frequent. At the time, I still lived at home, which offered some much-needed respite, and it was good to be able to escape for periods of time. But that didn't stop him from making me feel like a prisoner in my own home with constant threats of violence and humiliation. His most common form of manipulation was to threaten my family, stating that he would humiliate me in front of them or (worse) hurt them, which was unthinkable to me. This almost felt worse than the abuse I experienced myself. I was so fearful of him doing something to them, that it just felt 'easier' to bear the brunt myself instead. Despite how awful things were getting and how much his controlling behaviour was escalating, I didn't tell my parents anything. I really don't know why I didn't feel I could tell them, but I just felt that I couldn't bring myself to explain how bad things had gotten. I felt so much shame for allowing myself to end up in a relationship this bad. I had been so defiant about my relationship from the beginning that I had kept it secret from everyone, so much so that they had given up asking about it or how I was feeling. It actually felt easier to tell nobody than to ask for help. This meant huge amounts of secrecy and the hiding of bruises and marks on my body, which made me feel constantly on edge. For the twelve months we were together, it was the shame of it all that kept me silent. I was ultimately most afraid of him, but I was also deeply fearful of anyone finding out that I'd let myself get into such an awful position. And I was most ashamed that I was choosing to go back to that situation, time and time again.

Many people who haven't been through such an experience might ask why I didn't just leave. The answer is, because I was completely consumed by both love and fear, in equal measure, at the same time. I wish people understood that it isn't as simple as just walking away. What people who haven't been in abusive relationships often don't understand is that abusers aren't always bad all the time. I remember how comforting it was during my healing from this experience when someone said, 'If your abuser behaved to you at the beginning as they did at the end, you would never be with them in the first place.' I guess that helped me to rationalize that you don't start dating a monster. You start dating someone you believe to be lovely, but slowly the mask slips and their true colours are revealed, but so often by this point you're in too deep. And they can still have moments where they show you the person they were when you first met them. The person that you believed to be good and kind and loving. And so you cling on to those moments, desperately hoping that they will somehow magically return to being that person if you just love them enough. But what also keeps you there is the manipulation and control. They will often isolate you from your support network, like your friends and family, and make you believe that your relationship with them is all you need. It can be incredibly confusing and exhausting. As a sixteen-year-old who didn't know any better, and who desperately wanted to be loved, I was totally sucked in.

I tried to break it off multiple times, but so often this was met with threats of suicide or worse. I distinctly remember one occasion when he sat on the edge of a railway bridge, threatening to jump. I was screaming – terrified, helpless and totally traumatized by the whole experience. I've always thought of myself as a caring person, someone who genuinely wants to help others. How could I walk away from this person when he clearly needed me? And how could I ever live with myself if he did do the worst? On another occasion after I'd said I wanted to break up, he rang me at home literally hundreds of times without stopping, to the point that my parents had to unplug the phone from the mains. Despite being able to escape to my parents' house, I was always under threat and always under his control. Another time towards the end when I tried to finish with him for good, he even came to my parents' house and screamed in their faces, demanding that I came out and faced him rather than hiding inside, sobbing helplessly. I became scared to leave the house and developed extreme social anxiety, which I still suffer with to this day. It's horrible to write this blow by blow, as it almost seems unbelievable to me now that I didn't just turn around and walk away from him sooner. That's why understanding the mechanisms of abuse have been so critical in my healing from that experience. Figuring out the complexities of abusive relationships and the impact they can have on your mind has helped me explain to myself and others why it wasn't as simple as just walking away.

In the end, his actions worsened, and it got to the point where my parents decided to get the police involved. Things had simply gone too far, and by that stage the fear we were all experiencing was unsustainable. I remember speaking to the police for the first time and having to recount the details of our relationship in front of my mum. They'd come to my parents' house to ask us some questions and I sat shivering at the kitchen table, my hands in my lap, furiously chewing the inside of mouth with worry. Strangely, it wasn't the police being in my home that alarmed me, it was the shame that the secret I had kept for so long was out there, and that my parents had now been dragged into it too. And, to make matters worse, they now had to sit and listen as I explained exactly how bad things had really been for a long time.

The police listened to everything I had to say that night. I told them about all the times he had hit me, threatened me and my family, about the verbal abuse and emotional manipulation that had tormented me for so long. They were kind, understanding and visited my ex the next day to caution him but, if anything, this intervention made matters worse. You see, for many perpetrators of abuse, there are very few deterrents that work. They're not afraid of repercussions, so even a visit from the police is nothing to them. And in the case of my ex, it only made him angrier as he could see that this time I was serious about leaving for good.

I can still clearly recall the day of the attack. It had been a while since he'd last tried to contact me and – probably naively – I thought he'd got the message that I was really finished with him and there was nothing he could do about it. I'd started to feel more like me again in school (none of my friends had any idea what I had been going through so I could leave it behind me when I walked in each day). So while I was still incredibly scarred from our relationship, I finally felt a sense of freedom that I hadn't had in over a year. As I walked from one building of my school to another, I had to walk through the centre of town, which meant crossing a main road. I was with a group of friends, laughing as we carried our heavy backpacks stuffed with books. A car suddenly pulled up on the pavement right in front of me. It seemed so erratic that initially I thought someone had crashed, but before I had registered what was happening, my ex and his friend jumped out of the car, with what I remember to be the most menacing looks in their eyes. From the moment the car mounted the pavement to the moment his hand made contact with my face must only have been seconds, but it felt like I was paused in a TV show, with everything and everyone moving in slow motion.

While that moment feels so visceral, I can't actually remember what happened next. No sounds, no images, just a thudding coming from somewhere that must have been either my head or my heart. I remember that all I felt was complete bewilderment that my worst fears had become a reality and here I was for all to see: shamed, embarrassed and now unable to hide any of it from my friends. After those few seconds of complete stillness, I started to run. I don't quite know how I did it, but with tears streaming down my face I managed to get myself to the school gates where I collapsed into a heap in the arms of a friend who happened to be standing there. Words wouldn't come out, so nobody quite knew what had happened, but my body was in a total state of shock and all I could do was cry. I was quickly ushered to a teacher's office where I was able to finally calm down and recount the whole story. So much of that day is a blur of confusion and tears but one thing that I do distinctly remember was that in that moment, as I told my story to a teacher, knowing that my secret was out there for all to see, I felt that I'd hit total rock bottom.

With hindsight, you might be surprised to hear that I have many things to be thankful for from that day. Most of the abuse that I had experienced up to that point, like the majority of domestic abuse, had happened behind closed doors, so the possibility of a conviction would have been really difficult. So, although in that moment my worst nightmare became a reality, I am now grateful that my attack happened in broad daylight, on a busy high street, with plenty of witnesses. The second thing that I am so grateful for is that it occurred during school hours, which meant that, despite my protests, the school called the police and logged the incident. This meant I was one of the 'lucky' ones, whose case went all the way to court and resulted in a conviction.

On the day of the court case, I remember feeling as though I was going to pass out or throw up at any moment. It was a grey and miserable day, the kind where it never really feels like it gets light – pathetic fallacy at its finest. I barely had the energy to get out of bed, but I also knew that I'd waited for this day for months; as much as I was dreading it, I also hoped it would give me some kind of closure to the whole experience. Normally I would have taken great pride in my appearance, but I threw an outfit of drab colours together, with no real care for what I looked like. I had been so focused on the outcome that I hadn't registered what was going to happen that day and it was only when we arrived at court that I suddenly realized I might see him. Fear shot through my body like a lightning bolt, and it took every remaining shred of confidence to get myself out of the car and into the building. But that was just the tip of the iceberg. Nothing could have prepared me for the trauma that I was put through that day. I was a sixteen-year-old girl being forced to give evidence in court and, not only that, I was there to be cross-examined by a prosecutor whose job is to convince the court that you're a liar and your story of events is incorrect. One saving grace was that I was able to sit in a separate room within the court and give my evidence via video link. My parents weren't allowed in with me, so I was ushered in by a woman. The room itself was small and boxy with a Bible on a table to my left, and a TV in front of me that showed a live screening of the courtroom. As I sat down, the lady offered the Bible up to me to swear I would tell the truth. As the case commenced, all I remember thinking was that my dad had chosen to sit in the courtroom and watch the case, while my mum stayed with me outside the video link room, which meant that he'd be sitting watching my ex accuse me of lying about the whole ordeal. To this day, I still want to cry thinking about how he must have felt in that moment, how much anger and resentment he must have felt towards him, as well as towards himself for perhaps not doing his best at protecting me. It's one of those memories that lingers with you as real as the day it happened.

The cross-examination was something I was wildly unprepared for. I didn't have a private lawyer, and only met my prosecutor minutes before the case. They briefed me as well as they could, but to be honest it was all a blur until the moment I was confronted with the reality of having to retell what happened to me. I still remember the prosecutor essentially saying, 'I'm going to put it to you that this isn't what happened, and that instead you're making this all up.' I remember trying so hard not to cry or show weakness, to just stick to my version of events, but it was at this moment that the floodgates opened.

As I helplessly mopped up my snot and tears with the sleeves of my jumper, I felt so small, so helpless, like there was nothing more I could do or say, like I might as well give up.

When the guilty verdict came back it should have been a euphoric moment. I should have felt vindicated but there was no elation, or cheer, or even a glimmer of happiness within me. There was just total numbness, and I will never forget the silent drive home with my mum and dad. I just sat staring out of the window at the world passing by. I don't really know how my parents felt that day, maybe because I was so wrapped up in my own thoughts, but it did feel like a final line in the sand for all of us to be able to have some closure and move on.

I tried very hard to forget the whole experience once it was over. As soon as the court case was done, I did everything I could to push every emotion and feeling down into a small box and throw away the key. My school and my parents urged me to speak to a counsellor, but I saw that as bringing up all the pain and trauma I'd experienced. I just wanted to move on with my life once and for all. Of course, that isn't the best way to deal with serious trauma and, looking back, I don't think I realized how much the whole experience of abuse had affected me. I was a teenager who was desperate to fit in, and I wanted to channel all my energies into papering over the cracks and being as 'normal' as possible. Of course, everyone in my school had heard about what had happened to me that day and I caught girls who I'd never spoken to staring at me in the corridor. I felt so ashamed and so alone.

Thankfully the gossip soon moved on to something or someone else, and after a few weeks I felt like normality was resuming. People stopped giving me pitying looks, which I was grateful for, and my friends were as supportive as they could be without me sharing the true reality of what had happened. It just felt too painful to relive, and at the time I was still incredibly ashamed of the whole experience. I carried a lot of guilt and blamed myself; despite having lovely friends it felt too much to share this burden with them. Instead, I channelled my energies into rebuilding my sense of self, which had been entirely shattered into a million pieces. It probably wasn't until I was in my mid-twenties that I started to realize the depth of the impact that the experience of domestic abuse had had on me. The compounding trauma never really went away, I had just buried it so deep that it took near enough a decade to work its way out. Over those years, rather than acknowledging that my trauma was the result of being under my ex's control, I sought ways to take back control of my life in any way I could.

Over the year that we'd been together I hadn't felt the need to restrict what I was eating as much. I knew he fancied me so although I didn't change in body shape much, and I still watched what I ate around my friends at school, I wouldn't stress so much about what my mum was cooking and I'd even treat myself when we went out together. But after the case had ended, I felt completely lost and soon those old habits started creeping back in. It started with my food. As my life spiralled out of control, food became one of the few things I could really establish a sense of control with. I'd wanted to be smaller throughout my teenage years, and because for a while after the abuse life felt incredibly challenging, it was easy to control and manage my food intake each day. I'd learned bad habits from my teenage years, absorbing all the diet chat that took place at school, but it was after this traumatic experience that I doubled down on my efforts. It wasn't conscious, but it became a coping mechanism for me. When everything else felt so difficult, at least there was one way I could make myself feel even the slightest bit better. And, with the relationship behind me, and still feeling the immense shame that came along with it, I felt that making myself smaller would in some way make me feel happier and more desirable again.

In essence, I had gone from one restrictive environment to another. I was trying to heal the trauma and lack of autonomy I had experienced by exerting control over the things I could manage. In a strange way, dieting was a place where I felt safe. It felt like the only thing that I could really steady myself with. And coming from that toxic relationship, all I yearned for was safety. To have gone through what I did, so publicly, in a school where gossip was like gold dust, felt like the ultimate humiliation. So I reverted to the only survival method I knew. I controlled what I could and hoped that in making myself look a certain way, I would hopefully gain acceptance and validation from the people around me. In my mind I was on show for all the world to judge, so I had to work extra hard to perfect myself and rewrite my narrative. Although it might not sound like the most supportive environment by other people's standards, I was really grateful for the friends that I had at the time. I didn't really have 'a best friend' who was there for me during that time, but within my group of friends it felt as though one day this massive thing happened, and the next it was completely forgotten. Their coping strategy, like mine, was to carry on as normal and pretend nothing had happened. By not adding fuel to the fire, everyone's attention moved on to something else and I was just grateful for the anonymity that the passing of school gossip gave me. Time ticked over, and I continued my studies in a relatively uneventful way, opting after much deliberation to take a gap year so that I could audition for theatre schools.

Looking back, I now see that the relationship with my ex had all the hallmarks of a textbook abusive relationship. But at the time, I just felt so trapped. For a long time I still blamed myself, thinking that I must, in some way, have caused the situation to happen, another reason why I continued to punish myself with restrictive eating. But I've only realized this over the last few years, after going to therapy and doing my own internal work to truly interrogate and recover from the experience. As time went by and I slowly began to heal from the trauma of what had happened, I had this urge to share my story. I recognized that I had a large audience of women, many of whom had likely either been in similar situations or were perhaps still in them and feeling like there was no way out. I looked online for charities that I could support who were doing amazing work for women who found themselves in abusive relationships and came across Women's Aid. After reaching out to them and visiting their head office to find out more about what the charity was about, I knew that I wanted to do more than just support them financially. That was when the opportunity arose to become an ambassador for them; while of course it felt scary to speak openly about my experience, the fact that I could be saving women from going through what I went through was far more important than my own fear. Women's Aid are an incredible charity doing life-saving work. They have really taken me under their wing and taught me so much about domestic abuse; as a result I've become so much stronger. My work with them has been so fulfilling; in my ambassador role I've spoken in Parliament alongside Mel B to campaign for changes in policy, addressed the Labour party conference and visited women's refuges, which house the most vulnerable of women at risk of homicide.

Through working with them, I've learned that while each person's circumstances will vary wildly, ultimately there are patterns that many of these relationships follow, which worsen as time goes on. The longer you stay, the more likely it is that an escalation of actions will occur. On average, a woman is killed by a man every two-and-a-half days in the UK. And a woman is most likely to be a victim of homicide when attempting to flee a relationship. These stats really take my breath away, especially when I think about my then boyfriend's escalation of abuse, and what might have happened if I hadn't eventually had the courage to leave. It doesn't bear thinking about. And my heart breaks for anyone experiencing loss and grief through domestic abuse. To be able to now advocate for a charity that saves thousands of women's lives each year and to help raise money for their vital services makes me feel incredibly proud. I've also just taken on the role of being a board member for a women's refuge that houses over 100 women at one time, all fleeing domestic abuse. This work gives me the opportunity to meet women who find themselves at the rock bottom moment I found myself in all those years ago. It is a real 360 moment for me to be able to provide them with some comfort and support at what I know can be the most difficult time of their lives. Ultimately, this work is something I never take for granted, and something I hope I'm able to continue doing for as long as I can.

Deep down there is still a part of me that hopes that my ex has seen how 'well' I'm doing now – mentally, physically and in my career. It sounds a little weird, but I do sometimes have this need for him to somehow know that I've made something of myself, despite how much he tried to destroy me. In a way, the success I've had in my career and the work that I've put into supporting other women is partly because I've wanted so badly to prove him wrong. For every time he told me I was nothing and for every time he made me feel completely worthless, I've been able to show I am completely the opposite. And prove to myself just how far I've been able to come.

The toll it took

By the time I started sixth form it was so ingrained in me that I had to be careful about what I ate that it was almost second nature to restrict. I remember being so conscious of wanting to impress boys that I could think of nothing worse than actually eating in front of them. I don't know why this mattered, but I think I just absorbed what I overheard about how they felt about girls who weren't particularly slim. We had a sixth-form common room where biscuits were available each morning break time. I have a vivid memory of seeing them on the first day and experiencing a pang of anxiety accompanied by the thought, 'No, I can't have those.' I was so conscious of potential judgement and shame. Although it might sound absurd, this is just an indicator of how entrenched my anxiety around food now was. Although I'd love to think that I was the only one experiencing this level of anxiety around food and weight gain, I know it was very much the norm among young women at the time, and still is to this day. This example of what was going on inside my head at such a young age makes me feel deeply sad; I mean, who doesn't like biscuits?! And who has ever known a boy of that age care about what a girl eats?

While there was no official list of foods that were and weren't acceptable, there was a sort of unspoken rule that sugary foods were a no go. It wasn't as though anyone explicitly said that this was the case; there was no diet rule book I'd read and copied, I had just understood that to abstain was to appear as if I was somehow more desirable and classier for being holier than thou. It was almost a badge of honour.

The pivotal moment in my teenage years (or so it felt at the time) was my final year prom. I was eighteen and desperately looking forward to the freedom that the end of school would offer me. I should have been enjoying and embracing those final few moments of childhood, where you ready yourself for the big wide world, but instead I spent the weeks leading up to it obsessing over every piece of food I ate, and doing nightly rounds of sit-ups beside my bed, in the hope it would give me a flat stomach in time for the prom. I had this skin-tight silvery dress that I'd found with my mum in Debenhams. I remember the feeling of total elation when we went to try it on and the size was too big on me. When the sales assistant commented that I'd need a smaller size, I remember wanting to jump with happiness that I'd managed to make myself small enough to go down a size. And the fact that not a lump or bump could be seen was proof that I'd achieved what I wanted to. I did feel amazing on the big day, but as soon as the meal was served, I sadly poked it around my plate, knowing that eating would mean I might lose the precious svelteness that I'd felt when I'd arrived. And while I can absolutely see the madness now of avoiding food and alcohol on a night that was meant to be about celebrating the ultimate freedom of passing into adulthood, at the time the thing I cared about most was whether my tummy was bloated in my dress. Now I just want to go back and shake my younger self for missing out on the fun that could have been had at this time. And I know I'm not the only one to have made this mistake.

While lots of things about that evening were wildly predictable – someone got too drunk, someone ended up leaving in tears and someone inevitably fell out with someone – something was different that night. As someone who had struggled with relationships up to this point, to my surprise, I *was* popular with the boys that night. It wasn't that I was suddenly inundated with offers of dates, it was more that I experienced what I think I'd always dreamed of, which was to feel as if I belonged and as though people wanted to be with me. I remember feeling so happy that all my hard work had paid off. The sheen on the memory has of course since faded; I see now that this was just another moment that deeply reinforced the idea that I was only desirable when I was as slim as I could possibly be. And so, when I think back to that night, it now makes me so sad thinking about how distracted I was, and how much I thought that the peak of my happiness was being admired by other people.

Years later, when I was actively working to unlearn my unhealthy relationship with food, I spoke to so many women, of all ages, who'd trodden the same miserable path as me. It was so reassuring to realize that I wasn't alone and that my experience was depressingly similar to that of so many others. It was then that I saw how the focus on my body had absorbed way more attention than really anything else in my life at that time. Food, exercise and constantly thinking about my appearance was a huge distraction. It's sad to think what else I might have done or achieved, had so much of my energy not been wasted by such an all-consuming obsession. This period at school was clearly a formative one, and sadly instilled in me many of the challenging behaviours I'd have to unlearn as I began my later journey towards genuine good health. And yet, it's taught me so much other stuff too. About how these behaviours become so ingrained in us, how we go from not caring about what we eat, to then having that switch permanently changed, to thinking about *everything* we eat, and how the acceptance and validation of others becomes so much more important.

One of the most common things I say when I'm training people now is to always ask WHY. So often we just blindly accept ideas, such as being smaller is better, without really questioning why. 'Why do you want to lose weight?' 'Why do you think losing weight will make you happier?' 'Why do you feel unlovable as you are?' Sometimes these conversations are confronting and challenging, and I've become used to tears in my onboarding sessions. Because often, sitting in front of me, I see women who are treading the exact same path of self-hatred that I had been on, without really realizing that there was and is another way.

As I reflect on my younger years, what's undeniable is that even though I didn't have an easy ride, I feel lucky that I grew up before social media really took off. While the pressures felt intense in my time, I cannot imagine what young girls nowadays must be feeling as they navigate school with the ever-constant distraction of hundreds of thousands of people online. It has unfortunately made the pressure to look 'good' even more acute. And the opportunity for not just validation but also comparison and self-criticism doesn't just stop at your peers and classmates any more, it now extends to potentially millions and millions of people. What a terrifying thought.

As I've reflected, it's given me a real fire in my belly to help the younger generation break the cycle. I look at young women these days and I want so badly to tell them that they are beautiful, lovable, wonderful human beings regardless of how they look, or the dress size they occupy. I might have thrown away a lot of time and energy with my preoccupation with thinness, but I hope that this book – and the work that I now do – can stop others from following the same path.

My move to London

Between leaving school and going on to create my Instagram account, where many of you may have come to know me, there was actually a period of my life that I remember very fondly, when I felt totally free. After leaving school at eighteen I didn't have enough money saved to go through the auditions rounds for theatre schools, so I took a gap year, convincing my parents that I was absolutely going to be on the West End stage in no time. I got a job working in a pharmaceutical company to pay for my auditions and spent every day in a dark room filing pages of research for scientific trials. I was a glorified filer, but I absolutely loved the sense of adulthood it gave me. During that year, my relationship with food was still relatively restrictive but a little more stable, and while I hated that all my friends had gone off to university with all the fun and opportunities that that brought, I also had in mind the ultimate goal of training at a theatre school, and that kept me focused. That year felt like a time where I could just press pause on life and recover from the difficult few years I'd gone through. And on reflection, I'm grateful that it was a chance for me to really enjoy being at home with my family for a bit longer.

I began the audition process during that year, and it's safe to say I found it challenging at times. I'd always loved dancing, singing and acting, but being among some of the country's most hungry, talented performers competing for just a handful of spots at the top performing arts schools meant competition was fierce, and at first I didn't have much luck. Before starting my auditions, I'd envisaged walking into the room and the panel being stunned by my talent, instantly offering me a place.

I genuinely thought it would be that easy. The reality was there were thousands of other stagey kids like me who were all equally keen to take the few places available each year. I got 'no's from Arts Ed, Laine Theatre Arts and Mountview, the three schools I'd had at the top of my list, and by the middle of my gap year I was close to giving up hope. A nagging voice in my head kept telling me I just wasn't good enough. Thankfully, just as I was about to lose faith and extend the contract for my pharma job, I auditioned – just before the closing deadline – for Bird College, a performing arts school in South London, and was offered a place on their degree course. I genuinely couldn't believe my luck. I was going to live out my dream of training in musical theatre.

Moving to London felt like a dream come true for me. It didn't matter that I was in a tiny box room in Greenwich, or that there was one dingy shower for eight people to use. I would have lived in a tent if it meant I could train in musical theatre. I remember walking into my new flat on moving in day with my mum, and as soon as I met my flatmates I just knew that I was in for a good time. It was freedom, and it was *everything* I'd been yearning for. Even so, moving away from home felt like a huge deal and having grown closer to my parents following my experience of abuse, I did do the classic thing of bursting into tears the second my mum left. That aside, I was so ready to embrace being nineteen and living in the big city.

My fondest memories of my first year at Bird College definitely come more from the socializing I did rather than the training itself. From the very beginning, I knew I'd found my kind of people, and the fun we had together will stay with me for ever. When it came to the course, it wasn't that I didn't enjoy the classes (I did) but it was tougher than I ever imagined it could be. As someone with a history of disordered eating, and a challenging relationship with my body, what I hadn't come to fully appreciate is that I had stepped into an industry that was completely focused on physical appearance. The theatre world is full of diversity, except when it comes to body shape, and that's particularly true if you're a dancer. This fact was drilled into us from the very first day. During my first ballet class, I found myself standing in a room full of mirrors surrounded by beautiful, tall, slender girls with legs up to their armpits, and I felt my confidence dwindle immediately. I was sure that I didn't belong. I didn't have the traditional dancer's body; I wasn't long and lean, and I had boobs and a bum that seemed an anomaly in the room. All this meant that I felt I had to constantly prove I deserved to be there.

During my gap year I'd worked to relax a little around food, but despite the pressure of body image being drilled into us from day one, when I arrived at Bird College, I actually went the opposite way and totally threw off the shackles of dieting for a while. I think this was because for the first time in a long while I felt truly accepted by the people around me for who I was. Sure, I still stuck to some old wayward habits during the week, like only consuming a packet of Ryvita and butter each night for dinner for a spell, but I also partied hard, I mostly ate whatever I wanted, I slept in late and I ordered Domino's every Sunday with my flatmate Emily and would enjoy every single slice. It was as if all the work I'd done previously to try and fit in at school didn't matter any more, because I'd finally found people who truly accepted me. Body image certainly mattered within classes but outside, it felt like looking the part fell low on the priority list. If I had to say when I was happiest at college, it would absolutely be in that first year, where I finally achieved the freedom, both literally and metaphorically, that I'd been craving.

However, this did all come to a crashing halt at the end of my first year. Looking back, it was one particular conversation that made the momentous difference to my whole life path moving forwards. Even at the time, it felt huge. At the end of our first year, we were called one by one into a meeting with our head of year, where they looked at our marks in various disciplines like jazz, ballet and tap, and gave us feedback on how we were doing. After my peers had all come out looking pretty happy with their chats, it was eventually my turn. I was invited into the office where I sat opposite my very petite head of year tutor, who gave me a worryingly stern look. In as many words, the summary of my first year was that I lacked strength, I didn't have much potential and I was falling behind.

The sting of her words hit me like a ton of bricks. I knew I wasn't the best, but I didn't realize I might actually come close to failing my course. My passion for musical theatre was something that I wasn't going to let run away from me, and I immediately knew something needed to change. During this conversation, my tutor's word choices were interesting. It wasn't that she said it explicitly, but there was an absolute insinuation that being smaller would be helpful for my future career. She used words like 'stronger' and 'more supple' and whether she meant it or not, my brain went straight to the fact that my body had more curves than most of the other girls in my class. And suddenly, my brain clicked to the idea that perhaps the partying, and my diet of sweets and chocolate every night – no matter how fun – weren't going to get me any closer to my ultimate dream of being on the stage.

It was that simple. My slight period of respite from dieting and *not* being obsessively preoccupied with my body went out the window; in its place came a newfound focus to prove my tutor wrong by becoming everything I thought she wanted me to be. The version of me in the place I find myself today would love to have questioned why an industry that is so brilliant at celebrating some forms of diversity couldn't possibly accept me at the size I was. But I was young and naive, and I looked up to my teachers more than anyone else. So I nodded and listened, all while feeling a deep sense of shame inside that no matter how much I loved what I was doing, at that point, I wasn't good enough.

And so I set out on a new path. I left that room, walked home and immediately created my @cleaneatingstudent

Instagram account, to document my healthy lifestyle change, from waking up hung over and eating pizza for breakfast, to getting the body I thought I needed to fit the mould of a West End star.

My knowledge of what constituted a healthy diet at that point was incredibly limited. My only experience thus far of trying to lose weight was being incredibly restrictive with my food intake or doing the Special K diet and eating nothing but rice cakes. But with the amount of energy I needed to get through a whole day of dancing, those bad habits weren't going to cut it. I started to read up on nutrition and what I really needed to eat to a) build lean muscle so that I could be strong for my dance studies and b) drop body fat in order to look the part. The answer I came up with (after a very brief Google search) was that carbs were out, protein and (certain) fats were in, and that I needed to count both macros (macronutrients, which include protein, carbs and fats) and calories to monitor my overall energy intake. It seemed fairly self-explanatory at the time, and there weren't hundreds of thousands of social media accounts or blogs to look to for advice in those days, so a website with a basic macro calculator was my first stop, and from there I was ready to go.

I started eating smaller portions of protein and vegetables at each meal and taking pictures to document in my online food diary. It's actually laughable now how terrible my first foray into Instagramming really was. I remember one of the first images I posted to Instagram was a very unseasoned and dry chicken breast with some broccoli and sweet potato, photographed on a chipped plate with a sepia filter for a little bit of extra pizazz. I mean, culinary superstar I was not, but it did mean that I was making meals from scratch, and the online sharing aspect meant that I felt some level of accountability for sticking to my new regime. When I first started posting online, some friends made fun of me behind my back. I knew that there were a few people throughout my dance college experience who thought what I was doing was silly and that there was some bitching about me, but it didn't deter me.

I am, of course, acutely aware now that I simply replaced one form of dieting and restriction that I'd learned in my teenage years with another. Restriction can be dressed up in many ways, but the reality is that it was still calorie restriction in its most basic form. The difference for me was that because the foods I was eating were so much more nutrient dense and were perceived to be 'healthy', at the time I was totally oblivious to the fact that I wasn't eating enough and that my methodology was actually quite flawed. Very quickly, my weight started to drop.

After a few months of eating in this way consistently, my body had undoubtedly changed quite a bit and I started to get praise from my teachers. All the validation I'd been craving during my first year from my teachers and peers was suddenly being showened upon me in abundance, all because my body had got smaller. And with this validation came greater confidence in myself and my abilities, which meant that things started to finally happen for me in a way that they never had before. I got better roles in productions, I got asked to be part of extra pieces for shows and my results improved immeasurably. It wasn't as though my talent had drastically increased, it was just that I started to believe in myself, because other people were now seeing me in a different light. Needless to say, all of this confirmed to me at the time that when I was thinner, I was better.

While I thoroughly enjoyed my time at theatre school and would never want to bad-mouth the people who taught me, there were times when certain teachers definitely encouraged us to be smaller. It wasn't that they explicitly told us that we needed to diet (although shockingly, I have heard of this happening to other girls), but it was made clear that those of us with even a hint of curves should try to slim down. Because being thinner meant you had a better chance of succeeding in the cutthroat industry we all dreamed of entering.

It shouldn't have come as a shock to me that this kind of culture existed. As I mentioned at the very beginning of the book, one of the more challenging memories of my theatre school experience was being weighed on my first day. It was an achingly humiliating experience that left all the girls in my group solemnly gazing at the floor, even though it was a standard part of the audition process. We found out later, that when some girls in my year deviated from their original weight and were called to see the pastoral team, that our weights had been recorded that day. We all learned fast how much the number on the scales *mattered*. It meant make or break for many aspiring dancers. While dancing ability was essential, size mattered almost as much. There was definitely a part of me that, despite arriving at college in a normal, healthy body, felt that I wasn't quite small enough to fit the mould. So, when I managed to change my body and I did look the part, and when I started to receive praise for it, it felt like the ultimate success.

The reality is, I truly believed what I was doing was healthy. It just felt for me that to switch from the booze-filled fun and chaos of my first year, to the three meals a day of nutrient dense foods in my second year, was a huge and sensible difference, and I automatically assumed that I was doing things right. When many people around me were using what I saw as unhealthy methods to stay thin, like existing on fizzy drinks, cigarettes and sweets all day for energy, I genuinely believed that my protein shakes and homemade meals were worlds away. I simply didn't see that I had straightforwardly replaced one form of damaging restriction with another.

Making it

What made my lifestyle change a little different to just another diet was that I decided to document the entire process on social media. This was 2014, when Instagram had just burst into being as a fun platform on which people shared images of cute pets, beautiful sunrises and pretty (and not so pretty, sometimes, in my case!) plates of food. It was effectively an online scrapbook that you could share with friends, and you built a narrative of who you were through the little squares of your profile. It was nothing like the polished platform of today, where the line between people's real lives and slick advertising often feels invisible. It was messy and imperfect, but it was fun and it was different to anything that had come before it.

I'd initially started my page as a private account where I intended to use it to keep some accountability for my diet overhaul, using it as a visual food diary of sorts. It meant that I put a little more effort into the meals I was making, and it encouraged me to be more creative in the kitchen, which was a good thing as, despite my mum being an excellent cook, sadly her talent was not passed on to me and I really was terrible prior to that. I'm not sure where I'd heard the term 'clean eating' before making the page – perhaps on Instagram or elsewhere, but I felt it perfectly summarized what I saw as my objective: remove the 'bad' foods and insert the 'good' foods. At the time it felt totally unproblematic to think this way and nobody questioned it, so it felt like the right fit as a title for this new way of living. It's kind of like choosing your first email address. (Mine was sexy_bunny_girl@hotmail.com . . . clearly I haven't got much talent for choosing usernames.) But I was a busy theatre school student and had absolutely no idea of what lay ahead for the page, so I didn't think much of it or take it hugely seriously.

This came at the time where the likes of Deliciously Ella and Joe Wicks were emerging as big names and the promise of changing your diet, healing your body and somehow becoming a better person in the process too was so enticing to me. In noticing that they were building these amazing communities of like-minded people that seemed so encouraging and friendly, I slowly realized that I too wanted to connect with other people who were following a similar journey. Although I kept my page private for the first few months, the idea of opening it up to reach a wider community became more and more appealing.

In those early days, as some of you may remember, my page was mostly full of photos of chicken, broccoli and eggs. Lots of eggs! No real creative flare went into taking the photos, it was a cheap white plate from Sainsbury's, with nicely arranged (if quite bland) food on top, alongside a caption that explained what I was eating and a little about what I'd been up to that day. Over time, I felt that I lacked the sense of community I really wanted to get from sharing my journey. I didn't want to bore my housemates by talking about my new diet as they enjoyed their chicken nuggets and chips each night when we sat down for dinner, and so I slowly started to toy with the idea of making the page a more public and personal one, so I could connect with like-minded people. And so, after not much deliberation, as I sat on the bright orange sofa in our little Sidcup student flat, @clean_eating_student became @clean_eating_alice. And so was born the handle that I became known for.

The decision to make my page a public one was never about gaining more followers or becoming an 'influencer'. You have to remember that this was a time when that word didn't even exist yet, and the possibility of running a social media account as a career hadn't really been invented. My ambition came from a genuine place of wanting to create and engage with a community of people who could help motivate and inspire me, over anything else. What I didn't expect was that in the space of only a few months, I would see that following skyrocket, and my community grow to the hundreds of thousands.

At this point, I was still very much a theatre school student, enjoying the routine of ballet every morning at 8am, and the hustle and bustle of rehearsals and performances as second year pressure ramped up. None of my peers at college were aware of what I was doing online, and while the page was now public, initially I don't think anyone except my closest friends followed it. As we transitioned into our third year, the opportunity to audition for roles in productions and to get an agent was top of the agenda, and competition between students became rife. The reality of having to leave the college bubble and enter the real world of theatre was dawning on me, and I knew that if how I looked mattered this much while I was in college, it would only matter more once I left and was thrust out into the big wide world of open call auditions. So, while it wasn't my sole focus during that time, I enjoyed the escapism that continuing to grow my Instagram profile following provided.

There are few moments I remember more clearly in my life than when I got my first real job in the theatre world. I'd been seen for the audition a few weeks prior, and I did feel it had gone well. I'd smiled, picked up the routine quickly and actually enjoyed the whole process, which was rare for me in auditions. When my agent called to tell me that I'd got the job, I couldn't believe it. I stood still in total disbelief, unable to produce any words before bursting into tears (I've always been a crier). I was incredibly fortunate to get a year-long contract with the UK tour of *Annie the Musical* while still in my third year of training. I had to say goodbye to the comfortable bubble that was my college experience, leave the place that I'd called home for the last three years and pack my suitcase to head out on tour.

It might sound a little funny to say this, but I'd always dreamed of being successful in some way. From a young age I've never been afraid to go after things and shoot for the stars. So when this job came in, it was as if despite all the difficult experiences that theatre school threw at me, I had made it. I'd done something that just a few years previously had felt like a distant dream, and it felt so good. Not only was I leaving Bird College with my dream job, I had also made some of the best friends I'd ever had, and I'd built an Instagram community that was growing fast. It felt as though life couldn't be sweeter.

When I reflect on this time in my life, it's easy to see how this transition meant that I leaned more on my social media friends and followers. Leaving my friends and setting out into the 'real world' felt exciting and terrifying at the same time, and the community that I was growing kept me propped up and feeling supported, regardless of where I was in the country. Being on tour meant staying in a new city almost every week. There are different types of touring in the theatre world, with some shows spending long stints at venues, and others only spending a week at each location. We started our year-long journey in Newcastle, and after a rocky start of turning up at my first 'digs' to find a bed without bed sheets and a constant drip coming through the ceiling above me, I made the decision to make sure that year on tour didn't stop me from continuing to show what I was eating online.

I understand that some people might now see my life as privileged, and I know influencers can get a bad rap for 'not really working a proper job', but that year of touring was *hard*. The kind of hard graft that shapes you and makes you appreciate everything that you then do following it. We were performing eight or nine shows a week, constantly moving around to new locations and living entirely out of a suitcase, all while being paid £400 a week. It wasn't glamorous, but boy, did it teach me what a hard day's work was like! In addition to the demands of the show, I was determined to keep my community growing online, so as well as the clothes I needed for the year, I made sure I had my own plates and serving ware with me everywhere I stayed. (There was no guarantee that any of the places along the way would have the same style plates as me, and I wanted to maintain the consistency of my content style.) Despite an increased intensity of physical exertion with going to the gym each day, rehearsals and then one or two shows Monday through to Saturday, the reality was that during this time I kept my food intake exceptionally restricted. Being on tour is hard enough without trying to diet at the same time, but I just had this fixation with the fact that they'd hired me in a small body, and so I had to stay that way. Cooking from scratch wasn't always possible and so I became exceptionally organized, saving all my money aside from what I spent on accommodation to buy food and regularly prepping meals that I could take with me to the theatre. I also became incredibly familiar with the calorie content of certain foods that I'd buy on the go, and when my lovely castmates would buy sweets and treats, I was always the 'disciplined' one who watched what and when I ate.

It was around this time that I started to share more of myself on my page, and not just pictures of food. As my physique had changed, my confidence soared, and I enjoyed showing off my newly chiselled six-pack, taking great pride in the fact I looked so different to before I'd started to diet. At college I'd joined the local gym and found a new lease of life building confidence with my training. I was a real gym newbie, so at that time my workouts consisted of rotating around 10–12 exercises using weights, but for me it felt amazing. I honestly felt as though something had switched in me and I'd found a way of moving my body that I really connected with and enjoyed. The reality was that being on tour meant that I only had a little free time during the day to work out, as most of our time was taken up either rehearsing or performing in the show. Because of this, instead of just accepting that I was likely getting plenty of exercise from the show itself, I convinced myself that it wasn't enough and that I had to work hard to really carve out time to train. So despite finishing work at 10.30pm each night, I was up at 6am every morning to make sure I got to the gym. While this amount of exercise was in the realms of being problematic, in that my energy output was wildly different to the amount of energy I was consuming through food, this was when my love of fitness really grew and became a crutch. I used it to help with homesickness and missing my friends from college. You see, even though it was my dream job, touring can be incredibly lonely. I'd worked hard during my college years to build a stable support network of friends and family, but now I was lucky if I saw those people once every few months. So, in making my page more public and sharing more of myself, who I was and what I enjoyed, I started to really develop a bond with those who followed me, and it seemed that in return they felt the same.

After some time, I realized it wasn't just followers that I was getting attention from. During those first few months of the tour, I received not one, but a handful of offers from publishers who were keen for me to put pen to page and share my journey through a book. I wondered for a while if the enquiries were even genuine. At first, I thought it must be a scam of sorts. But when I received a message from a literary agent, I dared to consider if there was some truth to the messages, and when I googled the agent's name, the credentials they had shared with me seemed to ring true. Despite my following by this point being around half a million people, there was still a part of me who saw it as nothing more than an enjoyable hobby, something I did for fun. Of course, I'd seen people like Kayla Itsines and Joe Wicks soar to success with their books, but I didn't think I was anywhere near their level.

When I got the official offer to write my first book, I was sitting in my dressing room in Southampton, waiting for our evening show. It was a white, shabby space (as many dressing rooms are) with three tables in a row, all with mirrors and lightbulbs surrounding them. Next to me were my castmates Sinead and Anne, who I adored and who made touring such a special experience for me. I got the news via email and I let out an audible scream, quite literally falling to the floor. Both Anne and Sinead swung round to see what on earth had happened to me. I told them, through my tears, that I'd just been offered a two-book deal with a huge publishing house and was to begin writing straight away. At the time, in all the excitement, I didn't quite comprehend what writing a book would entail. It was almost as though with each new exciting moment of this Instagram journey, I just lapped it up, but the book was ultimately a huge shift. Here were publishers paying me a good sum of money for my expertise, of which I actually had very little. Of course I loved nutrition and fitness, but this was elevating me and positioning me as an expert, which I now realize, of course, I absolutely was not. But none of this bothered me in that moment, because I was young and ambitious, and I believed that everything was going to be okay. It was a life-changing sum of money for me, a life-changing opportunity, and I simply didn't feel at the time like I could turn it down. And so, in that tiny dressing room in Southampton, being hugged and cheered on by my two closest friends on tour, my journey to becoming an author began.

2. Where it all went wrong

It felt like I was riding high, achieving everything I'd dreamed of and more. Having been in such a dark place as a teenager, not only had I managed to make it to theatre school, but I'd gone on tour, finally had a body that people admired and complimented, and now I was getting recognized when I popped to the supermarket or to grab a coffee. In the space of just a few years my life looked and felt incredibly different, and I was so grateful for all that was happening.

As much as I was taking every step of the journey in my stride, when my Instagram account took off and my follower count kept increasing, I spent a lot of time pondering 'why me?' What was it about me that drew people in and made them interested? Of course, there was the obvious physical transformation. I had lost weight and my body had certainly changed. And, with hindsight and given how pervasive the 'thin ideal' was (and still is), I can understand that my followers bought into the idea that if they ate like me and trained like me, they might achieve the same results. But what started to grow was a feeling of being completely out of my depth. When the account was just a hobby, there was no pressure to do anything other than share what I wanted to share, but throughout that year on tour, as I signed with a manager and started to work with brands on various campaigns, I felt an overwhelming pressure start to mount. This was no longer a hobby; things were getting serious.

I can pinpoint the period immediately following my first book deal as a time when anxiety crept into my life in quite a big way. Not that I'm expecting pity. I should (and could) have simply held my hands up and walked away, because the reality was I was in no position to give people dietary advice. During that time, I was constantly waiting for someone or something to catch me out, for my success to suddenly shatter into pieces. In just a few months I had been parachuted in as the poster girl for fitness in the UK, with very little experience and only a basic personal training qualification to show for it. Despite some outward bravado, inside I felt completely bewildered by it all.

That isn't to say that I didn't love the excitement of what I was doing – I did. I mean, who wouldn't? While still away on tour, suddenly I was being invited to glamorous events and to do interviews for magazines. It was *OK!* magazine on the phone one week, and *The Times* newspaper the next. It was difficult to fit everything in – I remember finishing a show at 10pm one evening, driving down to London from Manchester (where we were performing), walking in a catwalk show for London Fashion Week as a fitness star at 10am the next morning and then driving straight back up to Manchester to do the evening show. The pace was relentless. Everything was happening so fast that it was almost impossible to not be swept up in the thrill of it all. But, aged twenty-two and fresh out of theatre school with very little life experience (and even less credible fitness experience), I did have huge pangs of doubt about going along with all the opportunities. And yet, I did. And I do hold a deep sense of shame for that.

The attention and 'fame' were surreal, overwhelming and addictive all at once. As my audience grew, my desire to be liked and to feel the warmth of social media validation increased. It was as if I'd somehow cracked the code of how to lose weight and people were coming to me as if I had all the answers. Of course, I didn't. But I was seen as the expert and I had to assume that role pretty quickly, so I could continue to ride the wave, despite my burgeoning inner imposter syndrome. This is perhaps where there started to be a divide between what I was sharing outwardly and what I was feeling inwardly. On the outside I was a happy-go-lucky, positive and dedicated girl who hadn't a care in the world, but on the inside I was riddled with self-doubt and worry about the pressures that came with having such a public profile and so many eyes on me. What had started out as an innocent side hustle had within the space of a year snowballed into something much more. It was no longer okay to just fumble my way through posting pretty pictures; I needed to assume an authoritative role on all things health and wellbeing. I didn't want to reveal any chinks in my armour, so I said nothing, and instead of asking for help or admitting I was no expert, I tried very quickly to accelerate my knowledge by booking myself on to various courses and reading as much as I could, so that I wouldn't be 'found out'.

And so, consciously or subconsciously (or perhaps a bit of both), I realized it was important to appear as if everything was okay. I'd built my platform by being the easy-breezy twenty-something who ate healthy meals and was always smiling. To put across anything other than that risked uncovering my growing inner turmoil and jeopardizing my fast-escalating career.

Writing my first book meant I had to juggle an intense schedule of doing the show while also writing all the recipes and content for the book. In the space of about six months, I had to write up and test eighty recipes, as well as pull together 20,000 words of accompanying text. Working on the book kept me up at night, but it was also something that I really enjoyed doing. Needless to say, the stress of producing it on top of my crazy working hours meant that my eating and exercise regime was becoming even more restrictive. The pressure of the book deadline, working in the show and trying to keep all my plates spinning meant that the only escapism I had was in the control I could have over my food and my body. There was something about being on tour and having all sense of routine thrown out the window that made me crave a sense of normality even more, and the only place I could get that was with my food and at the gym. So while my castmates went out drinking and enjoying each city we visited, I would head home straight after every show, have my pre-bed snack and then fall into an exhausted sleep . . . before getting up early to do it all again then next day. No one ever questioned my decisions, because it all seemed completely normal under the guise of being 'dedicated to the cause'. I remember so many of my castmates kindly commenting that they wished they were as 'dedicated' as me. But looking back, I feel I missed out on so much.

What was strange about this time was that losing weight and shrinking myself down was a fairly 'easy' thing to do. The formula was simple – once I'd grasped the concept of a calorie deficit (eat less, move more), my body responded quickly. What I struggled with though was the pressure to then *maintain* that physique in the long term. Once the high of achieving my 'goal' subsided, I needed to make sure that I kept my aesthetic. Almost all my 'success' was bound up in how I looked. I was known as 'Alice with the abs'! What people don't tell you about dieting is that if you keep inputting the same formula, it starts to work less beneficially over time. When you consume less energy for a prolonged period, your metabolism down-regulates; the formula that once worked decreases in its effectiveness. It wasn't that I gained much weight, I was just having to eat less and less to stay as small as I wanted to be. I began battling with my body on a whole new level. It was tough; I became hungrier, grouchier and more fatigued, despite trying harder than ever to stay lean. My body was screaming out that it needed more energy, but the thought of eating more filled me with fear. Gaining weight and going back to the body I'd worked hard to transform was not an option.

The reality is, I had very little understanding of nutrition, and even less experience in advising other people on how to approach theirs. I was trying so hard to make it seem as though everything was okay and that I had my shit together. And yet I look back now and realize how exhausting it was, constantly teetering on this precipice of being 'found out', fearing that it could all come crashing down on me at any moment.

To me, that's the problem with dieting. We see it as the path to this magical place, where changing our body suddenly solves any other issues we might have. By simply shrinking ourselves we believe we can achieve ultimate happiness. I shrank myself, and I felt happy for a while, but the body I'd slimmed down to wasn't one I could healthily maintain in the long term. It was quite literally firing all the signals – like extreme hunger, brain fog and fatigue – at me to show that everything wasn't okay, and I blindly ignored them all, because the pursuit of thinness was much more important than acknowledging those things. I'd become the fitness poster girl; I'd shared a journey that hundreds of thousands of women had bought into. I just couldn't face having to walk away from that, as awful as it sounds.

*

I want to pause here and take stock. I know that a lot of this might sound quite heavy and self-critical, but there is an important point to be made. Hindsight is a wonderful thing. It's difficult to unpick how much of this damage I was aware of at the time, and how much I only recognize to be problematic now with the growth and learning I've done since. While I carry a deep sense of guilt for the damage I may have done to my followers in terms of their relationship with food and their bodies, I also have compassion for myself, because at the time, I genuinely didn't know any better. I was myself a product of the wider context of the fitness and wellbeing world back then. The landscape was vastly different compared to today. Body positivity wasn't a phrase I'd even heard, let alone one I understood, and in my echo chamber, everything I was doing seemed completely normal. I didn't hear anyone question how 'healthy' what I and others were doing. The fitness industry was deep in the 'no days off' and 'no excuses' phase, and I fully believed that what I was doing was inspiring and aspirational. Behaviours that I now know to be deeply problematic, such as removing whole food groups from your diet and never allowing yourself a day off from exercise, were completely normalized. Without challenge, a lot of people, myself included, bought in to those toxic habits.

Nearly a decade on, I have the life experience that has allowed me to see clearly how much I was struggling internally. The world of social media has shifted dramatically since those early days. I and the many other people who ran similar accounts at the time simply didn't realize that we were perpetuating harmful narratives, that what we were doing was potentially damaging to hundreds of thousands of women. I was under the illusion that it was all about discipline and if I could only exert enough discipline in my diet and exercise routines, then everything would be fine.

I now find it difficult to reflect on some of the things I did back then, that I believed to be completely normal at the time. For example, I avoided almost all social occasions that revolved around food, in case I was tempted to eat something I didn't perceive to be healthy. I became the master of finding excuses and cancelling plans so I didn't have to answer any awkward questions about why I wouldn't have a slice of pizza or a glass of wine. I became so entrenched in eating from a limited range of foods that to venture away from that path was to step right out of the safety zone I'd created. I don't know whether I had a fear of the actual foods themselves, but I was certainly scared of gaining weight and what that would mean for my identity.

For anyone who has lost weight in the past, I'm sure you know what I mean when I describe the kind of halo effect you acquire from those around you. There are compliments and comments, and you feel showered with the warmth of approval that losing weight brings. So when it comes to sustaining that weight loss, the pressure is even more intense. If you deviate even slightly from the body you've been told is you 'at your best', you feel like the ultimate failure. I experienced this myself and as a result, I sadly developed an incredibly disordered eating pattern, as well as body dysmorphia. Even at my smallest, I wasn't satisfied with the body I inhabited. I would look in the mirror each morning, checking myself to see if anything had changed, and I never truly liked what I saw. There was always something that I would pick at, or feel self-conscious about, which just proves how even when we get to where we think we want to be, our inner critic is never truly satisfied. It was utterly exhausting.

For the first few years of my rising success, I only ever received positive comments about how I looked. I was told I had the 'ideal' body, or that I was 'goals'. There was never once an interaction where someone suggested that I might be underweight, or that I was too small. Not from my family, friends, agents, publishers or anyone else for that matter. That's why I so vividly remember the first time someone openly called out my behaviour and acknowledged it for what it was: disordered.

I was on a job in South Africa where I was filming a commercial for the South Africa Tourist board. It was an amazing opportunity, and something that I absolutely wanted to do, but it also filled me with dread as I knew I'd have two whole weeks outside of my comfort zone, away from my strict food and exercise routine. When the filming team and I arrived in Johannesburg, we were whisked straight into our first activity, which was a market tour. We had the opportunity to try the most incredible street food, and although the smell of it made my mouth water, I nibbled tentatively at each offering, trying not to draw attention to the fact that I couldn't face 'falling off track'. This pattern continued for the next few days. At each place we stopped to get food, I would scan the menu, searching for the lowest calorie option to eat. At one such restaurant, I ordered some biltong and a side salad, while everyone else ate the most incredible looking burgers. All the while I told myself that I was the 'healthy' one, when indeed the opposite was true. I didn't once miss a gym session or take a day off. I was missing out on the best parts of an incredible trip, all because the most important thing to me was staying thin.

It was during a dinner at a beautiful seafood restaurant in Cape Town that one of the team pointed out that I didn't eat very much. As we sat on two long tables, everyone else joyfully devoured the local delicacies and fresh fish that were served to us. Because of the so-called 'halo effect' that being 'healthy' can bring, instead, I found it completely normal to ask the waiter if I could please have plain white fish and vegetables only, something I'd done at previous dinners on the trip too. The comment wasn't said in a nasty way, nor was it meant to upset me, but it was an observation that stunned me for a moment. I swallowed hard, and my mind raced as to how to reply.

Up to this point, I'd existed in a complete bubble, where all I heard was that I was the healthiest version of myself. But I guess there was something about being on this trip, surrounded by people who all had such normal relationships with food that made what I was doing seem, for the first time . . . unusual. Although my real wake-up call came much later, I do vividly remember that dinner. It briefly jolted me from my belief that everything I was doing was completely okay.

I guess this is when thc smoke and mirrors began; the part of my journey about which I feel the guiltiest. Having been on social media for a while by this point, I knew all about the behind-the-scenes work that goes into creating a perfect image. Very few people *actually* bound out of bed and head to the kitchen to make a smoothie every morning at 5am. A lot of work goes into that 15-second video you see while scrolling. In my time online, I've interacted with some of the biggest fitness, nutrition and wellness stars, many of whom I can without doubt say were or are deeply affected by eating disorders but portraying a very different image on their social channels. With the ability to curate any narrative you want, nobody who follows you is really going to know if you really ate that piece of cake you took a convenient photo of yourself with. Or whether you genuinely did enjoy the takeaway pizza you filmed yourself taking delivery of. So it becomes easy to paint a picture of what you want people to believe, regardless of whether it's reality or not. And I absolutely played my part in this for a while.

You see, it was becoming more and more clear to me

that I needed to keep up the facade of everything being okay and projecting the healthiest version of myself. In reality, I was starting to be dishonest about what I was actually eating. As an example, if I posted that I was having eggs on toast for breakfast, often I'd end up removing the toast and just having the eggs and vegetables instead. Or if I was out for dinner with friends, I'd take a picture of their pizza instead of sharing the salad I'd ordered. It was an attempt to appear 'balanced' and 'normal'; I was pretending that I didn't have issues with food when the truth is that I did. I'd go on press trips or excursions where people I followed online would poke food around their plates, or skip meals intentionally, while telling their audience otherwise. It was as if we were gatekeeping the real reason we occupied 'lean' bodies, while telling our audiences it was absolutely okay to eat bread and ice cream. In hindsight, it was an awful time, and you'll be pleased to hear I have since very much distanced myself from that world.

When I think now about why I did it all, I am absolutely clear that I never purposefully wanted to hurt or harm anyone. I have to be fair to myself in that sense. But I also must acknowledge and take responsibility for the harm I perpetuated. I was selling a version of myself that people looked up to, when really my periods were becoming erratic, my hair was falling out and my personality and shine were fading, all because I felt I needed to remain small to be accepted and liked. I'm deeply sad for both myself and anyone else who got swept up in that falsehood. To this day I still feel a huge pang of shame about this aspect of my journey. That I essentially lied to people is a painful pill to swallow, and while to some extent I feel a sense of relief that I'm now comfortable enough to own my mistakes, it doesn't take away from the fact that they were deeply damaging and it doesn't make it any easier to accept that they happened in the first place.

First doubts

It was the day of my second cover shoot for *Women's Health* in early 2018, possibly the biggest single thing to happen in my career so far. I'd been working towards it for weeks, and all the excitement and nerves culminated in that moment. I was standing in front of a full-length mirror, staring at myself in a black leotard, my hair piled on top my head in an ornate plait, with big high heels on. I should have felt on top of the world, a million dollars, but despite all the 'hard work', including saying no to so many different foods and choosing exercising over spending time with friends and family, I still wasn't satisfied. Even though I'd been working extra hard in the run-up to the shoot, it was as if my brain wanted to seek out all my insecurities and amplify them.

Something just didn't feel right. *I* didn't feel right. I'd arrived at the shoot with all the usual nerves you might expect ahead of something as big as a national magazine cover shoot. But thrown into the mix was the feeling that I hadn't really earned this reward. I felt like a fraud, as though I didn't really belong. Put simply, my inner critic was screaming louder than ever before. Despite all the creeping negative thoughts, it felt easier to just keep smiling. Doing anything else would mean I wasn't living up to what people expected.

I felt that so much rested on the shoot. I was being given this incredible opportunity, but what had I really done to deserve it? What were people going to think of me? Had I gone too far in terms of how slim I was? Had I not gone far enough? I knew that I was small, toned and muscular, with visible rippling abs, but I also worried for the first time that maybe this wasn't what people wanted to see on a magazine.

To a certain extent, I'd lost my sense of self. As I got ready to have my pictures taken, I had to summon every ounce of energy to be the Alice I thought people wanted me to be. I'd become so wrapped up in the world of social media, followers and 'likes' that my true identity had fallen by the wayside. Much more recently, I've talked about this in therapy as I work to undo some of that damage, and I can see that I almost had to disassociate from myself in order to continue the fantasy. Deep down, I didn't believe I deserved any of what I was being given, but as each opportunity came in and as the jobs got bigger, I was too far in to just walk away and say I couldn't handle the pressure.

I had become an expert at putting on an act. (I was a

trained actress after all.) I breathed deeply. I was gracious and kind and smiley as the make-up artist worked her magic and I tried to push my negative thoughts away. I should have been grateful – I *was* grateful – but I was also lost with nothing to ground or comfort me. I focused on the task at hand by taking tiny sips of water and nibbling at a pre-made meal I'd brought with me. Of course, I couldn't fathom eating 'unknown' foods that I hadn't prepared myself ahead of a photoshoot.

Even after years of restricting myself and being booked to appear on the cover of a magazine to show off my body, I found myself feeling unworthy. Sometimes I *did* think I looked good, and I was often proud of parts of my body because I'd worked so hard on them and could see the results, but it was conditional. I had to be standing at a certain angle and have the right lighting to feel truly happy. Anyone else looking at me would probably have thought, 'She must seriously have no life to look that muscular.' It's so sad when you can't see what everyone else can; when you're so wrapped up in the pursuit of thinness that you can't ever imagine being totally satisfied. On that day, I still thought I could have done better, could have worked harder, eaten less, worked out more, not spent half an hour watching the telly while I munched on bland vegetables that morning. I always felt there was someone out there who was better than I was.

It should have been the pinnacle of feeling good. All eyes were on me, I'd had my hair and make-up done by experts, I was tanned, toned and had done everything in my power to feel my smallest that day, but despite everything, it didn't feel enough. The photographer snapped away as I sucked my stomach in, trying to find my best angles.

As the shoot progressed, I looked over to the monitor to see how the pictures looked in real time. It gave me a small feeling of control as I picked up on tiny things I believed to be flawed – a little roll of skin here, or a hair out of place there. They were all highlighted on the brightly coloured screen for everyone in the studio to pore over. I kept running over to the monitor asking them to change things. 'I don't like that. Oh no, that's not quite right.' I realize I must have seemed like *such* a pain, but it came from a place of massive insecurity. I'm sure these lovely people must have wanted to shake me and say, 'but you look amazing' and they *did* tell me I was looking great, but it fell on deaf ears. I just couldn't bring myself to believe them.

When the shoot wrapped up, I was mentally and physically exhausted. When you're operating from a place of such low energy, even the smallest tasks can take it out of you. Putting on a good show of pretending I was the happy bouncy Alice everyone knew from social media had left me drained. I was tired and hungry as well as depressed that instead of feeling on top of the world, I simply didn't. I kept wondering, when would I?

It was all a bit of a wake-up call. I'd done everything to look my best that day – most of it the opposite of what was genuinely good for my health – and I still didn't feel good enough. Why? I had worked almost to the point of collapse, and I would still see pictures of other women and think, 'she's got longer legs than me' or 'her stomach is flatter' or 'her arms are more toned than mine'. That's the danger of social media; no matter how good you look and how good you feel, someone else can come along and make you feel totally rubbish. From an outside perspective, I'd probably done a great job, but when the shoot was over I felt tired and deflated.

Although I could have slept for days, I headed out to celebrate my exciting day with friends, something we'd planned in advance as a little celebratory meal. I hadn't been able to tell many people about the shoot, but my closest friends at the time were those I was working out with at the gym and I felt able to confide my news in them. In hindsight, I think that dinner was probably what got me through the shoot. I loved the idea of spending time with friends, but in reality, I often struggled with it as socializing so often revolved around food, which meant I was always fearful of 'falling off track' or eating off plan. My usual stance was to avoid most social things as it felt safer. This time, however, was a chance to forget the pit of loneliness in which I found myself and instead focus on doing something 'normal'. I pushed the boat out and allowed myself a margarita pizza and a glass of prosecco, and I remember the feeling of true happiness when I finished it all. Of course, I made sure to take a picture of my dinner and upload it to

Instagram, to ensure my followers knew I enjoyed a 'balanced' lifestyle. Nope, no eating issues here. Look at me enjoying alcohol and cheese! What I didn't mention is that despite having a lovely time, after finishing the pizza, feelings of guilt started to creep in and I left the meal early. Of course, my excuse was that I needed to get an early night and be fresh for the gym the next day. Needless to say, I didn't share that detail with my audience. And so, the charade continued.

One thing which makes me sad about that period of my life is that my laser focus on things like the *Women's Health* shoot meant I was often selfish. Thinness for me was in fact totally wrapped up in selfish behaviours. It wasn't that I intended to be selfish, but to stick to my many rules and regimes, I had little room left for anyone or anything else. Most of my social interactions were walks or gym classes with friends; energy burn was the only thing that made me feel I could justify socializing. What I struggled to admit then – but am able to say now – is that I was incredibly lonely.

During my time at theatre school and when I was on tour as part of *Annie*, I'd had tons of people in my life, whether because I was living with them, or sharing a dressing room with them every day of the week. I was surrounded by great people and that meant that however disordered my eating was becoming, I was never as isolated as I was when I moved into my own place in London. Moving provided the perfect environment for me to start shutting people out to focus on myself.

I talked myself in to believing that living alone was what I wanted (the reality is that it was just another way to exert control over my environment without outside interference), but week by week, month by month, my circle got smaller. Without realizing it, I became chronically lonely.

My friends probably did think I was a bit weird leaving so early that night when we'd gone out for pizza. Or maybe even a little rude. Years later, I spoke to one of the girls who was there and explained how I'd been feeling at the time. She listened patiently and then said that she'd had no idea, and that I'd managed to hide it all so well. It was incredibly cathartic for me to have that conversation with her. It helped me to understand some of the self-sabotaging things I used to do, such as cancelling social plans, things I hope I've now moved on from.

Despite finding the shoot day difficult, I did feel a lot of excitement in the run-up to the *Women's Health* cover coming out. It wasn't that I thought I looked amazing, I still experienced a lot of nerves in that respect. But I saw it as the ultimate proof that I'd made something of myself. It feels rather silly to admit, but part of me thought back to when I'd walked out of that courtroom as a teenager, a shell of my former self. I'd turned my life around completely, and that gave me a huge sense of personal accomplishment. I am a highly motivated individual, but I'd be lying if I said a lot of my motivation to succeed, particularly in those days, didn't come from trying to prove those who had doubted me wrong. I thought back to my ex, to the friends I'd left behind at school, to the teacher who sat me down in that first-year review with the pitying look, and the people who judged me when I started sharing my meals online. I've since learned that the sweetest success comes when you do something truly for yourself, but I knew no better then. At that point, my success was very much framed by how much I could prove to other people how well I'd done and how much they'd underestimated me.

When the magazine came out, I received thousands of messages congratulating me on my success, mainly from the women who bought into Clean Eating Alice and loved everything I stood for. As far as I can recall, there weren't any negative comments off the back of the shoot. I just got lots of lovely, kind people saying nice things. What that reinforced, therefore, was that it was so worth staying extremely lean. Being showered with praise felt amazing, and I was on such a high I didn't want to come down from it. In my mind, my body as it appeared on the cover of the magazine represented success. That was what mattered.

The reality of what people were seeing and how I was really feeling were very different though. I found myself swept up in a world that was both exhilarating and terrifying, and somewhere along the way I'd lost my sense of who I was. Maybe I *was* this fitness guru who should be congratulated for working so hard to become society's idea of physical perfection. But maybe I was just another pretty white woman, who was trying to sell an idealized version of what other women want. To be slim, to be liked, to be successful. I fitted the mould, but it was an almost entirely unfulfilling one, one that came at the expense of my day-to-day happiness.

I hope I don't sound too 'woe is me' here. While I think it's important to be honest and share exactly how I was feeling, there is also a huge part of me that acknowledges that I must take responsibility for my damaging actions, and I very much do. I think my point is, it's so easy to get swept along in life, rarely questioning your true intentions or feelings because it's easier to go with the tide than against it. And that's exactly what I did. As the praise for my work swelled, I swelled with it, and so I bobbed along, while desperately treading water underneath. And, as anyone who's tried to tread water knows, it eventually gets exhausting. A wave or two might lap over your head, but it's very possible to get in too deep, and even be at risk of drowning.

And that is the point at which I found myself when I entered Emma Cannon's clinic in 2018.

3. How it got better

Anyone looking at me from the outside when I was at the height of my 'success' in 2018 must have thought I had made it. I had accrued an incredible Instagram following of over 600,000 and I felt like a 'somebody' at last. With that came exciting brand collaborations, invitations to incredible events and opportunities out of my wildest dreams. The world of social media success can be a crazy one, and my feet barely seemed to touch the ground as opportunity after opportunity came in. I flew first class to New York with Gap, I partied in the Hamptons, I attended movie premieres, I released a clothing collection with Primark – I even got to interview Louis Theroux. Surely I was living every twenty-something's dream? I had worked hard and sacrificed a lot to carve out my career and for a while I convinced myself I was happy with everything I'd achieved. Then came a moment that made me rethink everything.

I had gained a big following, but the reality was that my body was suffering for it. I'd been so distracted by my increasing workload, my gym routine, my clients and writing my next book that for quite a while I totally overlooked the fact that my periods had stopped. It wasn't like I just missed one. I think I honestly forgot they were supposed to come monthly, and I vaguely took it as a blessing that they no longer did, as I'd always suffered with them. After a while I did start to worry though. One month passed, and then another, and the health anxiety within me grew as I became concerned about what might be causing it.

After multiple GP appointments, two gynaecological scans and endless pregnancy tests, nobody had the answers as to why I'd lost my menstrual cycle. I was fobbed off with options of going on the pill, or having the coil fitted, neither of which seemed like a sensible option for me at the time. I'd met Paddy, my wonderful fiancé by this point, but I knew that hormonal contraception wasn't something I wanted to be on (for fear of weight gain, would you believe). So after much deliberation I turned to other, more left-field options.

One sunny autumn morning, on the recommendation of a friend, I found myself sitting in the office of renowned fertility specialist and acupuncturist Emma Cannon. Emma's office was like a shabby chic living room, adorned with mismatched cushions, crystals and beautiful patterns on the walls that changed as you made your way through the room. On one wall there were photos of babies. Not just a handful of cute pictures; this wall was covered from top to bottom with gorgeous, happy babies, all of whom, Emma told me, she'd helped to conceive.

We sat down at a large, round table in the middle of the room, and Emma handed me a form. I duly completed it, fully believing I was a very fit, very healthy 25-year-old. All the tests I'd had and all the prodding and poking hadn't offered up a single reason as to why my periods were MIA, aside from a misdiagnosis of polycystic ovary syndrome (PCOS), which offered little relief and even fewer answers. Emma sat down at the table and flicked through my notes. She then began asking me a series of questions. 'How was I sleeping?' 'What did my tongue look like?' 'How many bowel movements was I passing?'

As I sat there, feeling confused by the direction of the questions she was asking (did this have anything to do with fertility, I thought?), she leaned forward slightly and fixed me with a kind look. 'Darling,' she began. 'You're too thin and you're doing too much exercise for your body to have a period right now.' She said it so frankly and matter-of-factly that I was uncharacteristically stunned into silence. I had no idea what to say back. No words came out of my mouth. But she'd spoken in such a maternal way and with such kindness that I had to believe her, even though I didn't want to.

What she was essentially telling me was that, by severely restricting my energy intake over a prolonged period, my body had stopped the production of hormones needed for ovulation, so I was no longer having a period each month.

I inhaled deeply and felt my face flush red, as if someone had read my diary and discovered my deepest darkest secret. It had taken Emma just minutes to look beyond my super-healthy facade and smiley demeanour and see the real me: a girl in her mid-twenties who was completely exhausted and devoid of any inner light. I wanted the ground to swallow me up. Emma very gently assured me that this wasn't the first time she'd seen someone in my situation, and that it wasn't a helpless case. She'd seen many women like me, all so distracted by the pursuit of thinness that they'd neglected one of the most vital health functions a woman can have. This made me feel both sad for those other women, but also relieved I wasn't the only one.

Emma said she was very used to seeing women going through life using contraceptives, and having no idea anything was wrong because the contraceptives simply masked the problem. It was only once they stopped taking them that it became clear things weren't as they should be. I have always been – and continue to be – a huge advocate of contraception, so please don't read this as me suggesting you should stop taking them if they are working for you. Everyone should choose what is best for them, and it's also a conversation that should be had between you and your doctor, as each case will be different and it's important to ask questions first before making rash decisions. But I am so grateful that I decided to come off mine. It was as if I could sense something wasn't right, and I needed to give my body a chance to let me know.

The combination of Emma's diagnosis, and the kindness with which she delivered it, and my anger at myself for treating my body so badly for so long brought me to tears. Deep down, I knew that the way I'd been living wasn't sustainable. That consultation with Emma was truly the turning point for me. As tears flowed down my cheeks, splashing into my lap one by one, I realized I was also crying because I knew that if I wanted to have the thing I yearned for more than anything else in the world, which was to start my own family one day, I would have to say goodbye to the underweight body I had sacrificed so much to achieve. I had a choice to make. I could continue down the path of restrictive eating and overexercising and maintain the body that had afforded me my career and a huge social media following. Or I could take a step back and allow myself to gain some weight, in the hope my menstrual cycle would return and my health would improve.

I will never forget how amazingly Emma comforted me that day. She spoke with the same nurturing voice that my mum uses. Whereas other people – like Paddy and my family – wanted to support me in my journey, Emma came from a more objective and removed place; she had the authority of an expert while also delivering the information as if she was a friend. Having dealt with similar situations before, she knew all the right things to say to calm me down. She was firm but fair, explaining that if I didn't change my lifestyle, I was going to end up potentially doing more damage and affecting my bones, my hormonal health and my chances of having children in the future. It was in that room that I knew I was at the beginning of a grieving process. The choice was hard but obvious. Was being applauded for my thinness worth the risk of never being able to have children? Of course not. But the thought of having to gain weight and be judged for it was also terrifying. All the same, to this day I am grateful for her advice, and I credit Emma with changing the course of my life.

A new relationship with food

Following my meeting with Emma, it wasn't as if I clicked my fingers and things magically fell into place overnight. Far from it. But that conversation made me see that change was necessary, which was a hugely important first step.

I'd become entrenched in my unhealthy habits over the course of several years, and it was extremely difficult to undo them. I had to unlearn my strict rules around food; the ones which dictated that certain types were good and others totally off limits. The ones that meant I avoided delicious croissants on a Sunday morning with Paddy, or a dessert when we were out for dinner with friends. Yes, some foods are naturally more nutrient-dense and contain fewer calories, but that doesn't mean we have to eat them *all* the time. There was so much that I'd indoctrinated myself into believing, that even starting to unpick it all was challenging.

One of the first things I did was get rid of my scales

and ditch the obsessive calorie counting. I think deep down I'd known that these external metrics were ruling my life far more than they should have done, and when I'd made up my mind that recovery was the only option, I knew that they had to go. In the past, I'd always sought out advice when it came to how I should approach my training, my diet and everything health-related. I wanted confirmation and validation that what I was doing was okay. But by this point I'd recognized that instead of those people (coaches, nutritionists, etc.) helping me, it was perhaps creating more of a confirmation bias that my low energy intake and high energy output was acceptable. This needed to be *about* me, caring *for* me.

I was so attuned to the calorie content of most foods that I didn't stop thinking about calories entirely, but at least I wasn't actively tracking every single one I consumed. I worked on incorporating more rest days, and filling my time with things that genuinely made me happy, like a lazy Sunday morning in bed rather than being at the gym for 8am. I had to start trying to be kind to myself, perhaps for the first time ever. That meant prioritizing all aspects of my health: how well I slept, how my mood was, whether I had a libido or not – and not just thinking about being slim and seeing that as all that mattered.

But as I took those early, tentative steps towards a new relationship with food, I encountered a whole different challenge: binge-eating. My experience chronically affected me for over a year, and it was absolutely debilitating, a form of self-harm almost. I would eat and eat and eat, and afterwards I would spend days feeling unwell and uncomfortable and promise myself I would never do it again. But the urge always returned and before I knew it, I was rifling through the kitchen cupboards once more. The self-loathing I felt was intense.

While the bingeing was (in part) me rebelling against the food rules I'd followed for so long, a lot of it was also me needing some sort of self-soothing while I went through a major readjustment of my lifestyle and values. Where exercise and abstaining from food was my default before, binge-eating became the new mechanism I used to regulate my emotions as my body changed and my identity shifted.

At the time, I didn't feel able to talk about my problem online. While discussing my changing body came relatively easily, bingeing was something I battled with privately. I wanted to be liked by my followers, and it seemed important to keep my content palatable and relatable. My changing shape was one thing, but explaining that part of the reason I'd gained weight was that I was struggling with an eating disorder? I could hardly say that! Eventually, I lost interest in exercise, in sharing my meals, in showing up online, full stop. In all honesty, I felt pretty much done with the whole thing. I had spells of feeling like a complete fraud. Instagram thrives on positivity, and I could not have been further from that place. I posted less, unable to muster the same energy I had for it at the beginning and unwilling to use the same smoke and mirrors. I'm unsure whether my followers initially noticed a big shift, but the reality was that while I was still figuring out what recovery looked like to me, I just couldn't pretend to be okay or act as if everything was 'normal'.

I knew I had to learn how to stop the bingeing, and I eventually started work with a therapist to help me do just that. I was lucky to be able to see a therapist, and I wish there was more readily available help for those with eating disorders, many of whom struggle for years and years. Something I learned through therapy is that binge-eating most often comes from a feeling of lack of control and the need to numb and self-soothe. Having controlled my food and training routine meticulously for so long, trying to let that go was petrifying. As my body began to change, I was wrestling with the fact that I was moving away from a place where I felt 'safe'.

Thankfully, with my therapist's help, the debilitating pendulum swings between bingeing and restricting started to slow down. As the pandemic hit and all of our worlds became more confined, I used my time to establish a long-lasting vision of health for myself. I really wanted to regain a regular monthly menstrual cycle and a positive relationship with exercise whereby I allowed myself adequate rest and a nourishing and balanced relationship with food. Underpinning all these things was my mental health. During the pandemic, when I had no access to a gym and felt less able to walk for hours on end each day (which I'd done a lot during my restrictive routine), I had an opportunity to almost start from scratch again with my health, and to prioritize how I felt rather than how I looked. I created a plan for regular home workouts, and got excited to make delicious, wholesome meals with Paddy, while also discussing what dessert options we might go for. It was as if, slowly but surely, I relearned how to genuinely become more intuitive with both my exercise and the food I was eating.

I can only speak from my perspective and tell you what my therapist taught me. I can't advise other people what to do. But for me, it was important to be able to separate my emotions from my reactions. If I wanted to binge, I would give myself a moment to process my thoughts and emotions first. I would stop and ask myself what I was feeling. Was I stressed? Was I tired? Was I sad? I would write it down to get it out and then, if I still wanted to eat, I would. But nine times out of ten it did help, and I wouldn't. I also used the five-minute rule: if I wanted to eat something, I would wait five minutes and if I still then wanted it, I'd have it. Sometimes even that small separation of time will help your brain rationalize whether eating is something you genuinely want to do, or if it's just a reflex. Both these techniques have worked well for me. They mean I can eat one biscuit now and put the rest of the packet back; I can have two slices of toast instead of ten.

I must admit though, I still sometimes have wobbles. I've even reached out to coaches and asked for their help to become smaller again, suddenly believing that things would be better for me if I got my old body back. I would rather be honest about that because I would hate for anyone who is struggling with something similar to think it's been a walk in the park for me. Things *do* get better, but it can be a slow process. Whenever I miss that feeling of being 'skinny' or put myself down for eating 'unhealthily', I remind myself what my old approach almost cost me: my health, my friends, my social life, arguably my sanity; and if I'd continued on the same path, who knows what else?

I still have therapy today, and I still have times when I do really need that help. This book is all about raw honesty, and so I must admit that I still have the odd binge day even now. It's become a weird coping strategy that kicks in when I'm feeling stressed, overwhelmed or anxious. It happens a lot less than it used to, and I've become much better at recognizing my triggers, but it's sadly not banished from my life completely yet. One day I hope I will be able to say that my days of disordered eating are totally behind me, and I am doing everything I can to make that happen.

Binge-eating is so often misunderstood, in that it's frequently used colloquially to describe people simply indulging until they're very full. That is not binge-eating. Binge-eating is a compulsive, insatiable drive to eat that isn't deterred by fullness. You eat and eat and eat until you feel physically sick, and even then, sometimes you don't stop. Those who have experienced the binge–restrict cycle will also appreciate that it doesn't mean overeating all the time. Following a binge there is an awful, overwhelming guilt, which can then lead you to overly restrict your food . . . and the whole pattern starts again. It's surely time for binge-eating to be dragged out of the dark, shameful cupboard it's been hidden away in for so long. It's a serious condition that needs to be acknowledged. It can be every bit as destructive as other eating disorders, but for some reason, it doesn't get much airtime.

If you are struggling with an eating disorder, please do seek the support you need and deserve. The charity Beat estimates that around 1.25 million people in the UK suffer from some form of eating disorder, but research suggests that around 46 per cent of anorexia patients fully recover, as do 45 per cent of bulimia sufferers. With the right help and support, that could be you.

Over the year or so that it took me to get from an intensely restricted diet to – eventually – a kinder, gentler approach, there were certainly signs my health was improving. I was sleeping better. I felt less fatigued. And I was genuinely enjoying eating a wide variety of foods again. But there was still no sign of my period. Many months had passed and I was beginning to really panic that I'd done so much damage to my reproductive organs that it might never return. After working on all the things Emma had suggested, I was keen to start the next phase of treatment, which was acupuncture, to see if that would help. After my first session, I went on to a work event and suddenly my stomach started to bloat. I remember it so vividly because I had to loosen the tie on my dress, as this unfamiliar sensation came over me. After experiencing it for around an hour, I had to excuse myself from the event and leave. I headed home and sat on my bed, feeling those old, familiar signs of sore boobs and a slight ache in my lower back. I woke up the next morning and there it was – a bleed. I had never been so happy to get my period. My clever, beautiful body had healed itself and I had never felt more proud of it.

Setting an example

It was during this time, not long after my pivotal meeting with Emma, that I made another huge change in my life: to change my Instagram handle. It might sound trivial to anyone who wasn't plugged into the wellness industry back then, but this shift was immensely symbolic of what I was going through in my own life at the time. I had built this whole brand under the name Clean Eating Alice, but as I began my journey of recovery, I started to see big red flags in being associated with and promoting the concept of 'clean eating'. When I created my Instagram account, I just didn't give it much thought. I imagined that only my friends and a few others might see the page, and so the name felt quite insignificant.

But the clean eating movement did indeed start to grow, and alongside it the negative connotations of what 'clean eating' meant became more apparent. I now understand entirely how problematic it is to label foods as either 'good' or 'bad', or 'clean' and 'unclean'. This binary approach to nutrition is so damaging for our relationship with food and by using that title, I was contributing towards thousands of women and girls believing that they needed to pursue a 'clean' diet in order to be healthy. While I wasn't fully aware of this at the time, there was a specific moment that started the ball rolling, towards me moving away from the name and everything it represented.

In 2018 I was away on a press trip in Greece with a fellow fitness blogger. It was an amazing trip, where we stayed in a beautiful tiny village on the Island of Tinos, where rows and rows of picture-perfect white houses lined the coastline. One morning I awoke to my phone receiving message after message of friends checking in to see if 'I was okay'. I was so confused – had something happened? I quickly read through them and realized that there had been an article printed in the *Daily Mail* that was less than kind about me. In as many words, it lumped me together with a handful of other leading 'wellness' influencers suggesting that we were the cause of an increase in eating disorders.

I was horrified. I remember staring at my name and just wishing and willing it not to be true. My horror turned to tears, and I felt this overwhelming sense of guilt that was incomparable to any guilt I'd experienced before. This was a wake-up call for me. While I never set out with ill intentions, it was unfathomable for me to carry on from this point as normal without recognizing the impact of my association to clean eating.

This was easier said than done though. I'd built this whole brand off people recognizing me under the name Clean Eating Alice, and it was a huge risk to step away from that moniker and almost start afresh. I discussed the pros and cons of it all with my team, and it didn't take long for all of us to come to the conclusion that changing my name was something that had to happen. Although the decision felt like an easy one, I was simultaneously filled with worry as to whether my audience would unfollow me or stop engaging with my content. And I did lose followers. But to this day, it is without a doubt one of the best things I've done, both for myself and my audience. It's helped me to broaden who I am and what I believe in. It felt like an evolution that enabled me to build a new life, free from the disorders that had defined me for so long, and able to work on undoing the impact of the problematic things I'd once promoted.

It wasn't just my handle that needed to change either. Everything about my approach to my body and my health had just been flipped on its head so I knew I needed to stop sharing photos that focused on my body too. Over the years I had mastered the art of getting glammed up to take a picture to post, making it seem as natural and candid as possible. But those days of perfecting my tan, hair and make-up and holding my breath in front of the mirror for hours on end are long gone now.

I stopped sharing workouts that called out specific body parts. Gone were the workouts that 'shredded your abs' or 'inflated your glutes'. I completely altered the way I spoke about exercise and how our bodies respond to it. My language changed and I built a new narrative that was worlds away from the 'no excuses' approach I had previously taken, not just for myself but my followers too. And I've worked to stop myself from seeking validation from strangers on the internet. Instagram is a visual platform, so there is no getting away from the fact that I still need to share content that has me in it, but my Instagram handle is now Alice Liveing and my clothing choices, angles and whole approach have really shifted away from 'the who' (me) towards 'the what' (what value I can add to help people see past how they look). I also really emphasize that my experience as a personal trainer has far more value than what I look like.

I rarely get comments on my body any more. No one really admires my abs or my arms, and I'm okay with that. I guess how I'd hope to be seen is that I'm just 'normal'. I admit that sometimes there's a part of me that thinks my life (and business!) might be easier if I had a body that was more lean and muscular. I'm still inundated weekly with paid advertising for fitness programmes with beautiful, perfectly conditioned women at the forefront, driving the idea that if only you trained like her, you'd look like her. In those moments, it's so important to bring it back to the WHY. Why am I doing what I'm doing? Why have I continued with it?

The truth is, I harbour a lot of guilt from my early days on Instagram and how I presented myself to the world. I didn't ever set out to hurt anyone, but I know that along the way, by default, I did. I feel responsible for causing people to develop unhealthy relationships with their bodies, food and exercise. That is why this book is so important to me. If I can put some good back into the world for those people who were affected by the image I naively put out there, I will be very happy. I was playing the part of someone I thought everyone else wanted me to be, and I lost myself in the process. Therapy has helped me to realize that, and I will be forever grateful for it. I can now rationalize and recognize that I was a part of the problem, but I also know that I wasn't the *whole* problem. I was a smaller piece of a much bigger puzzle.

Take back control

Nowadays, I have completely changed how I approach social media, both as a creator and as a consumer. Over the last four years I've routinely culled accounts that make me feel worse about myself. I do it all the time now. Why would I want to see things that make me feel miserable when I have a choice not to? We all have a choice, and I would encourage everyone to do the same, if they feel like social media is harming them.

When I did the first round of unfollowing, I wondered what had taken me so long. I know it may sound a bit odd, but I felt a real sense of freedom afterwards, knowing I didn't have to subject myself to content that I found triggering. I made a conscious decision that I would never live my life solely through social media again. I have made it just a small part of who I am rather than the whole of me. I limit the time I spend scrolling now and, most importantly, I question everything when I open any social media app.

The main things I ask myself are:

Do I feel better or worse about myself when I see this post?
Does it make me feel I need to change myself in some way?
Do I question the validity of it?
Am I comparing myself to this account in some way?
Is seeing these images bringing me joy or making me sad?

When I started viewing social media from the perspective of a discerning consumer, I reduced its ability to manipulate my thoughts and behaviours. Doomscrolling became a thing of the past and so did that nauseous feeling I'd get when I saw something that really bothered me. Ultimately, you and I hold the power when it comes to what we engage with and it's up to us to decide who we do and don't follow. We need to take ownership of how we consume content, because no one else is going to do it for us.

While there will always be many aspects of the online world that concern me, there are things I love about it too. When you start to look away from the picture-perfect influencer accounts and allow other types of bodies into your feed, that can be really beneficial. When I did it with my own Instagram, I can't tell you the difference I felt in myself. I didn't leave Instagram thinking, 'Oh my god, everyone looks amazing. She is beautiful. Her life is beautiful. She's so happy . . . I wish I was like that.' I started to appreciate other women's bodies for all that they are and how gorgeous they look. Thank goodness we are seeing more plus-size models and more diversity in advertising, film and TV too.

Question everything, and if it doesn't feel right, unfollow. It's the only way. My number one rule now is to only follow accounts that are uplifting or teach me something valuable. End of. I no longer worry about offending people by unfollowing them because my self-esteem is in a much better place now. Give it a go yourself. It feels bloody amazing.

4. The new 'me'

Breaking away from the person everyone believed I was took a lot of work. I felt like I was stuck in a bubble, where I knew who I was deep down, but it was still a huge challenge to distance myself from the phoney image of myself I'd created on social media. Recovery is not easy. It required a deep amount of self-awareness and self-confidence; even today, I couldn't say I am 100 per cent clear of it.

I'm a realist when it comes to recovering from eating disorders and excessive exercise. I'm now in a place where I feel quite neutral about my body. It's neither amazing nor terrible; I just exist in it. Sometimes I might have days when I feel great, or I wear an outfit and think, 'Wow, I look a million dollars in this.' And some days I might be on my period and feeling bloated, or I might have had a few drinks the night before and be a little worse for wear and speak negatively towards myself. I experience both ends of the spectrum but having the ability to bring my perception back to that neutral centre, and knowing that my feelings will all pass eventually, and that my worth, happiness, health and success don't have anything to do with how my body looks . . . that's empowering. I'm also able to question that pesky voice in my head, the one that tells me I'm looking a certain way. As a wise person once taught me: 'Thoughts are not facts, learn to question them rather than accepting them to be true.' So on those days when my brain decides to tell me something less than lovely about how I might look that day, rather than listening and accepting it, I challenge those thoughts and override them.

Looking at clothes differently

I hope I'm not making the whole process seem as though it was all rainbows and butterflies. It has been really hard, and some things have been far more challenging than others. One thing I've especially struggled with on this journey has been no longer fitting into clothes I've previously worn and loved. One dress in particular stays in my mind. It was short and navy blue, with feathers around the bottom, and I loved it. I wore it to my first ever film premiere and I remember feeling absolutely amazing in it. But when another event came along that the dress was appropriate for, I stepped into it and tried to pull it up, and it wouldn't reach past my hips. I was shocked; I didn't think I'd changed *that* much. I didn't cry, but I did feel torn. It was a complete juxtaposition of emotions. I so wanted the sensation I'd felt when I first wore that dress, with my old body. But I had to rationalize my thought process and realize that the body I was in now afforded me so much more life, fun, happiness and enjoyment than one silly dress could ever bring.

Most women know the feeling of dismay when one of their go-to outfits doesn't fit them any more. It's a trap so many of us fall into. The day I tried on that blue dress obviously wouldn't be the last time I would struggle to fit into old clothes. I knew it would happen more frequently over the subsequent weeks and months. I had to find a way to accept that deeply uncomfortable, triggering feeling. To learn to try and challenge that internal voice – and override it.

Having spoken to many women about weight gain and diet culture, I've learned just how common it is to get attached to clothes. They can have huge sentimental meaning, whether it's the top you wore for your eighteenth birthday, or the dress you splashed out on for your best friend's wedding. It can be hard to let those things go, especially if they represent a time when you were slimmer or felt at your best. A lot of us will hold on to an ancient pair of jeans that fitted us when we were at our smallest 'just in case'. Or there's a dress that will hang and hang in your wardrobe, because you're going to wear it again at *some* point, when you feel slim enough. Regardless of how arbitrary and pointless they are, we attach so much meaning to our clothes and the numbers on their labels.

I've spoken to a lot of women who hold on to their pre-baby clothes, even though in doing so, they're only punishing themselves. Instead, they should be celebrating the fact they've grown and nurtured a child – may be even multiple children! The expectations we place on ourselves are mad. Understanding that our bodies will change throughout our life is so important. At the height of my Clean Eating Alice days, it felt like a badge of honour when I went into a shop and could confidently pick up the smallest size, knowing it was going to fit me. I've since had to change my outlook and learn that clothing sizes mean nothing compared to genuine health and fitness.

I don't own any clothes from the slimmest stage of my life any more. This is me now; I do not plan on going back, and that's an important line to draw in the sand. As I've gradually updated my wardrobe, I've only bought new clothes that I really like, that make me feel amazing. I invest in good-quality options that will last and see them as an extension of the work I put in to being comfortable in my new body and all the positive things it has to offer. That said, I also have to promise myself to try my best not to see the numbers or measurements of any items I own, and instead always prioritize dressing my body in comfort and style. I know that as I age, and as I go through various life events like perhaps having children, and going through the menopause, my shape will change. When that happens I'm going to give my body the grace and compassion it needs rather than criticizing myself at a time when the focus really needs to be elsewhere. I really hope that in reading this book, you might find the courage to do the same.

On this path of finding my style again in my new body, I realized that I needed to feel special and buy things that I felt comfortable in. And in doing so, I enjoyed really finding my fashion flare. Those who follow me on Instagram will already know that I love fashion, but I genuinely believe that my new affinity with clothes and with creating beautiful outfits stems from no longer caring about the dress size – it's no longer the ultimate benchmark of value. Instead, I think about how clothes make me feel and what I genuinely love wearing rather than what shows my body in its 'best' form. In fact, my fashion journey has been quite a joyful one, opening up new opportunities for me to celebrate my body rather than rail against it.

One of the things that this process has taught me is that sizes don't mean anything. Over the last couple of years, my dress size has varied by four or more different sizes depending on the clothing brand. It can also depend on the cut and whether I want to get something oversized or tight, for example. Ultimately, I'm just not precious about it any more and I care so much less now because I have a vision of how I want to look in clothes, and that's far more important than simply squeezing into the smaller size because it feeds my ego. These days, my approach to buying clothes is to ignore the numbers completely. Instead, I work on finding the right styles, cuts and fits that suit my shape, regardless of what size they are. Numbers and measurements are different wherever you go, so choose a size that feels and looks good on your body, because you deserve to feel fabulous. Life is too short not to.

And isn't it crazy that we prioritize so many things over comfort when it comes to choosing outfits? I cannot tell you how many times I've been to weddings or events and someone's said to me, 'I can't eat today because I've squeezed myself into this dress and there isn't an inch of room left.' Wedding food is often amazing. Why would you want to miss out on it?! I'm in the process of shopping for my own wedding dress at the moment; my number one stipulation is that on the day I'm able to breathe in and out fully, sit down and eat my wedding breakfast *and* have multiple glasses of champagne and be comfortable. That's way more important to me than squeezing myself in to something slinky, only to feel horribly uncomfortable on what's supposed to be the best day of my life.

Clothes should be the casing we wear to feel good. They're a representation of who we are, how we're feeling and what image we want to portray. For a long time, I hid my changing body in baggy clothes, tracksuits and leggings. There's nothing wrong with those kinds of clothes and I still wear them regularly as well as lounge around in them most weekends, but I denied myself the chance of feeling good in anything else because of the mindset that told me that my body wasn't good enough. The reality is that all of us deserve to feel wonderful in whatever we choose to wear, and while that will look different to each of us, the most important factor is that you are wearing what makes you feel your best.

No more guilt!

No matter how comfortable in my skin I am now, there are still moments where I am reminded of how I used to look and that can be hard. I try to acknowledge it and process it as best I can. Building a personal toolkit of things that help you challenge those moments is so important. For example, I sometimes remind myself about how much I enjoy my training now, compared to the exhausted obligation I experienced in the past. I recently posted a picture on Instagram that I took on Boxing Day a couple of years ago. It made me so sad when it came up on my Timehop, because it was the first Christmas I'd allowed myself to eat and drink what I wanted . . . great in principle but the reason I'd taken the photo was to shame myself into dieting again because I was convinced I looked terrible. I was bloated and feeling very 'bleurgh' (that's the only way I can describe it). Even though I'd simply been enjoying a more normal Christmas, I was making myself feel bad for it. I decided to post that photo publicly because it showed me how far I'd come, and I hoped it would show people that I was human too.

The response was overwhelming. It was both saddening and reassuring to hear from people who'd done exactly the same thing themselves. In those moments when we feel so alone in experiencing such deeply challenging emotions, there is something comforting in hearing that others know what you're going through, because they've been there themselves.

Thankfully my recovery has continued since then, and last Christmas was the best one I've ever had. My progress felt palpable and I had so much fun. Paddy and I got engaged on the 19 December; following that magical moment we had about a month of non-stop celebrating. I ate whatever I wanted and felt the most free and comfortable I have done in years. And amazingly, not once did I turn to a mirror and think, 'Oh, I've gained weight.' Not because I stopped myself from doing so, but because it didn't even cross my mind. I was high on happiness, on love, on all the wonderful, joyous things that I'd deprived myself of, and it felt incredible to know that this moment that I'd dreamed of for so long wasn't impacted by negative thoughts that I should or could have looked different. It seemed like the most momentous progress.

I know some people will disagree with me on this, but I think it's unrealistic to expect people to come to a place of complete self-love straight away, where they spring out of bed each morning and look in the mirror and absolutely love every inch of their bodies. I'm not saying it's not possible; some people absolutely do achieve it. But for most women I've spoken to, and in my own experience, self-love is something you aim for, while self-acceptance is something you can practise every single day – even when we've eaten a larger than normal meal or enjoyed a week of ice creams every day on holiday. I firmly believe that working *towards* body-image acceptance is one of the most positive steps you can take.

On the days when I wobble, I repeat to myself, over and over for as long as it takes, that I am loved, kind, happy and so much more than just a body. My family and friends don't love me any less because my body has changed, so why should I? The vessel we inhabit needs to be treasured. It's an amazing thing to get to have children, to thrive in our chosen career, to age and to wear a bikini in our seventies if we so wish. Approaching our bodies with acceptance and kindness is the only viable way I can see to bypass the relentless diet dogma that we are bombarded with, and instead live life to the fullest.

Acceptance looks like waking up each day and simply saying that you accept who you are and where your body is right now. You don't have to love it. You just have to say (out loud if you can) that you are accepting that this is the body you inhabit, and you're not willing to diet yourself smaller if it's going to be to the detriment of your health and wellbeing.

I feel lucky to now be able to enjoy my food and training routine in a healthy way, without constantly worrying, or feeling as though I'm not doing enough. My happiest moments over the last couple of years have been when

I've had total freedom and felt comfortable with my body, for example when I've been out for nice meals with Paddy or my friends, ordering exactly what I want from a menu rather than spending ten minutes evaluating the calorie content of each dish. Nowadays, I pick whatever I feel like eating and can say confidently, 'I want this for a starter, this for my main and that for dessert', which feels such a huge step forward. I can look in the mirror after a big meal and think, 'I'm not this terrible person. I haven't gained weight or become less lovable because I've eaten a dessert with my dinner. And I don't have to exhaust myself in the gym tomorrow to make up for it. If I do choose to exercise tomorrow, it will come from a place of wanting to feel the joy of moving my body rather than it being a punishing routine that starts the whole depressing cycle again.'

Body acceptance and neutrality isn't the same as body positivity, which has its own origins and advocates who rightfully own that space. Instead of placing such a heavy focus on physical appearance, body acceptance is all about recognizing your body's abilities and non-physical characteristics. It's why I believe it ties in so perfectly with exercise, and why I have totally changed my social media content to reflect the shift I've made in my own mindset. There is so much content online that implies that the purpose of exercise is to change your body, and that your sole motivation to work out should be to improve the way you look. But what I want to do, and what I strive to do every day with my platform, is to highlight all the other amazing benefits of exercise. It could keep you moving and motivated until you're eighty! And that's so much more beneficial than simply picking up and putting down exercise when you've got a holiday or big event coming up.

How we feel about our bodies, and how we choose to move them are intrinsically linked. Through learning about this and understanding the importance of language in how we relate to exercise, I have had to adapt the terminology I use when discussing exercise on my platform. Rather than 'burn' 'earn' 'blast' 'tone' and 'destroy', I've switched to more positive and empowering words like 'strong' 'capable' 'dynamic' 'energized' and 'powerful'. Even these smaller, almost imperceptible shifts play a part in presenting exercise in a whole new light. Now I approach it as one of the best things I can do for my health and wellbeing rather than something that exists only to make my body look a certain way. This is what I hope I project online and in my classes too.

When I get there, then . . .

One of the most important lessons that I've learned over the course of my recovery is that there is no such thing as 'getting there'. I think many of us could do with totally unlearning the idea that when you lose weight or see a certain number on the scales, then you'll finally feel happy/good enough/lovable. Chances are you won't ever 'arrive' at that magical destination.

There's a false promise that everything's going to be fine when you reach a certain weight; that all your other problems will simply melt away. While some people will genuinely benefit from losing weight, many others find the vicious cycle of dieting an impossible merry-go-round to get off and it can evolve into a lifelong problem. I do think that dissecting the genuine motivations behind a fat-loss goal are important, to ensure that there's not too much hope that everything in your life will be somehow better once you are slimmer.

I wish I had the secret formula for body acceptance. None of us are alone, and all of us have so many similar touch points in our stories and journeys to where we are now. For me, the big question was, 'How can I learn to love and accept a body that is different to the one I thought was me at my "best"?' I don't think there is one answer, because diet and body issues are so complex. But as someone who has worked incredibly hard at trying to accept myself regardless of how my body looks, I now find myself in a relatively consistent place of peace.

I also want to caveat everything I've said so far by acknowledging that I'm still in a small body. I am in no way suggesting that I am that much bigger than I was before, nor can I speak for those who occupy that space. There are already some incredible influencers who are doing amazing work in the body-positive space for curvy and plus-size people, and I would never want to speak about something I don't have experience of. I am talking from a purely personal perspective, as someone who has gone from being underweight to where I find myself now.

I know that my journey is similar to so many other people's; as I've said previously, it is in realizing we are not alone that we can start to take steps towards recovery and be shown that there is another way to approach health and wellbeing.

As women, we are conditioned into believing that smaller is better and thinness equals happiness, popularity and finally feeling 'good enough'. But I cannot tell you how many women have starved themselves down to their ideal size and they still don't feel okay. Surely that is proof enough that thinness *won't* bring you everything you're dreaming of.

On some level, many of us know that it's not great to feel so awful about our bodies day in day out, but our insecurities convince us that if we shrink ourselves and stay small, life will be better. A thin body is more often than not praised and envied. A lithe figure is so often equated with success, even if that person is punishing themselves daily by eating as little as possible. The irony is that we dedicate so much time, energy and headspace willing ourselves to be slim, in order to achieve happiness, that we miss out on many of the genuine joys that life has to offer.

I am passionate about shattering those decades-old

myths. I've been that person. I've poured a lot of honesty, time, energy and love into this book so I can hopefully stop others from going down the same well-worn path I took. I hope it's clear that there is another way; one that is so much more fulfilling, sustainable and rewarding.

I feel fortunate to have come out the other side of what was a very difficult and damaging experience, with fire in my belly and a desire to stop others from going down the same depressingly predictable route. I know it's a bit of a cliché, but I want people to realize they are so much more than a number on a set of bathroom scales or on a clothing label. Please believe me when I say there is an alternative. Life should be about saying yes and doing more, and that doesn't have to mean feeling out of control or being completely 'unhealthy'. When we let a more restrictive life go, we let more joy in.

When I'm triggered by something, like an old photo of myself for example, I sometimes have a wobble. But I also now have the ability to check myself and ask questions that challenge those inner demons. I've worked hard to focus on what's important to me. It's not about never having those thoughts again, it's about learning that they're not facts, and they shouldn't dictate how I live my life. By letting go of those negative old thought patterns, I allow more space for positive ones to come in.

My happy ending

When I met Paddy, back in 2017, I immediately felt that he was different from anyone else I'd ever known. Our first date was in a little coffee shop on the Kings Road in London. Even that detail is a strange reminder that I was actively avoiding anywhere to do with food or alcohol at that time, so going for coffee was one of my very few options for seeing people socially. I was still in a very vulnerable place dating wise, and I found it difficult to let people in.

When I think back to my earliest memories of him, the overwhelming one is an impression of kindness. As we chatted, the conversation flowed easily and naturally. We had grown up in the same area, although we had no mutual connections, and we enjoyed lots of the same things. At the end of the date I remember this unfamiliar sensation of warmth, like I'd just spent time with a good friend. At this point I had some very complicated food issues, and though I did my best to disguise them, I think that it made our early dating life difficult. I rarely wanted to eat out at restaurants, I didn't drink alcohol and I didn't ever stay out late. My world was so small, and it revolved entirely around my food and training schedule. Our second date was a meal that I cooked at my flat, which meant I could have full control of the food we were eating and how it was cooked. It's an amazing feat that he stuck around and put up with this so early on.

Alongside my difficult relationship with food, I was in quite a dark place mentally too. I'd become so isolated because of my pursuit of thinness that I didn't really know how to receive love, or how to let people get close to me. There were instances in those early days when I was difficult and even tried to push Paddy away, because that seemed easier than letting my guard down. I wouldn't speak to him for days because he'd done something small to upset me, or I'd go completely cold and act as though I'd been too busy to message him. Deep down I didn't want to be behaving like that because I really liked him, but I didn't know how to override my protective mechanisms. I've worked a lot on this in therapy since. Essentially, it was my way of sabotaging the relationship because I didn't believe I was good enough for him, and that now makes me desperately sad.

While a lot of people played important roles in my recovery, what Paddy was able to do for me – and what I wish someone could do for every person out there – was to reflect the good qualities I had back at me. He was able to show me the things I didn't see in myself, like that I was genuinely likeable, funny and kind. I found it hard to recognize these aspects of myself because all my energies had been focused on *how* I looked, not *who* I was. He was able to give me what I needed when I needed it most. Slowly but surely, and with time, my guard started to come down, and I began to long for the joy and fun I saw Paddy having with his friends. I wanted it for us and, more importantly, I wanted it for myself. I'm so fortunate to have met someone with the patience and kindness to do that for me. I never in my life believed that at thirty years old I'd be engaged to someone as wonderful as him. I hope (and am confident) that we will have a wonderful, happy, healthy life together. And when I reflect on my turbulent previous relationships, I am overwhelmed with joy that I now have someone as brilliant as Paddy as my future husband.

Meeting Paddy was a major catalyst for me to start to heal even more. It was like a seed being planted. Something needed to change because I had been so full of self-hatred; suddenly here was someone who genuinely loved me for me. Receiving unconditional love was a very important step in me then being able to show it to myself.

What our relationship has also taught me is that attraction runs much deeper than being about how you look. I'm sad that so many of us prioritize our appearance over who we are when it comes to dating. If you're reading this and putting any of your life on hold because you're not the size, weight or shape you want to be before you meet the right person, I hope reading this helps you see that numbers aren't what bring you happiness. There is no reason to wait. You are already so deserving of love. All of us will change throughout life because of hormones, holidays, pregnancy, illness – you name it. And no one should have to spend the rest of their life worried about how worthy they are, or how much someone is going to love them, because they aren't at peace with their physical appearance. Of course, initial attraction has its place, but if you find yourself with someone who prioritizes your appearance over the things that really make you special and unique, you have to question whether that relationship has the ability to go the distance.

I truly, truly believe that the least important thing about my and Paddy's relationship is how we look. Sure, I love getting dressed up and going out in a nice outfit, and I'm sure he thinks I look great. But when we are at home on the sofa and I'm in my pyjamas looking quite dishevelled, that's actually when I feel I'm most loved.

Where I am now

While it might sound like Paddy was my knight in shining armour, that's not exactly what I mean. Yes, he helped me on this journey, but it has been me who has dug deep through every difficult day. This is my journey and despite the ups and downs, I'm so glad it has brought me to where I am now. Ever since I was a little girl dancing around to Celine Dion in the kitchen, moving my body has been a huge part of my life, whether dancing as a child and a teenager, or lifting weights as an adult. Even after recognizing that I spent years pushing my body in the wrong way, these days nothing makes me happier than when I'm moving my body in the right way. Since qualifying as a trainer, I genuinely get so much joy from helping others to feel the same.

I remember when I started to get clients at the first gym I ever worked at in London. It was a small boutique gym in South Kensington called Lomax, and it was there that I learned what being a personal trainer was all about. It meant getting up at 5am every day, doing heavy lifting for each session as you set up your client's weights and then tidying everything away for them afterwards, as well as prepping your day's programmes for each client. But what I didn't expect of this experience was that I'd love it as much as I did. I never intended to be a personal trainer in the long term. I'd always envisaged going back to musical theatre at some point, but during that year I flourished in confidence and really found my calling.

It wasn't that I was the best trainer. I still had so much to learn, but that was almost what was so enticing for me, plus the fact that I really enjoyed connecting with my amazing bunch of clients. I've always loved one-to-one connection. I'm not great in big groups, but there was something about each hour I had with my clients where they got my undivided attention, and I cared about them all so much, from the very first session. My passion for coaching grew, and I booked myself on to course after course on everything from mobility to pelvic floor function; I was so hungry to learn more and to be able to impart that information to my clients. What started out as something I'd thought I'd do for a short period while I finished my second book and took a breather from the theatre world, actually launched the passion for coaching that I still have to this day. And it's this exact passion that has kept me wanting to share my expertise, even after becoming jaded by the more frustrating aspects of the fitness industry. After leaving Lomax for the prestigious Third Space gym in Soho, I really found my flow as a coach. I was surrounded by some of the best in the business, some of whom I continue to learn from.

When gyms closed because of the pandemic, like everyone else, my training was limited to what I could do from home. But that didn't stop me from sharing my love of lifting weights. Soon after the start of the first lockdown, I was deeply missing coaching my clients, and so I started to offer live classes via my Instagram. The response was incredible and what it gave me in terms of confidence in my coaching skills was a huge bonus. It really saved me at a difficult time when so many people were struggling, and it helped me see that I could reach thousands more people through an online platform. Rather than being able to only coach a handful of people each day, I could reach thousands. Not long after Give Me Strength, my app and my passion project, was born.

I cared a lot about my app being different to anything else that was out there. Of course I wasn't reinventing the wheel, but I wanted to make sure it had my stamp on it. My message was (and remains): it's not about getting a six-pack or becoming the leanest version of yourself possible. It's about following a structured, solid, evidence-based training programme that's going to get you (and keep you) strong. *And* you can have fun, learn new skills and challenge yourself along the way. Most importantly, it really doesn't matter how you look, or if you're 'good' or not. The focus is giving it a go and feeling good in yourself. I believe wholeheartedly in my approach, and in sharing my love of strength training with others, while not focusing on the physical transformation side of things. It's about celebrating all the other benefits that exercise can bring, such as how much of an uplift it can give you mentally, how it can improve your self image, improve your quality of sleep and lead to better cognitive function.

As I come to the end of Part 1, I'll admit that there have been times when writing this book where I've had tears streaming down my face. It hasn't been easy to go over and regurgitate some of the more challenging aspects of the last ten years. But I am so happy with where I am now. I think it's so important to share all the different elements that have led me to this point and to see how far I've come.

Last December I booked a photoshoot to capture some new images for the app and my Instagram. In complete opposition to any photoshoot that had come before it, the night before Paddy and I got a Dishoom takeaway (my favourite). I made the conscious decision to do the exact opposite of what I would have done in my toxic past. I chose to recognize that my body was exactly where it needed to be for the shoot. Happy, healthy, functioning as it should be. And I cannot tell you how much of a full circle moment that was for me. As I stood on set the following day, the lights warming the chilly studio slowly, I looked around with a deep sense of gratitude for everything that I'd done to get to this place. Standing there, with every ounce of confidence in the world, smiling the biggest, cheesiest smile and feeling truly amazing.

All the bumps in the road, the mistakes, the learnings, *and* the happy moments led me to that and have made me the coach and the person I am today. Although I'm happy with where I am now, and proud of myself for getting here, there are certainly moments along the way that I wish I could have avoided. My hope is that by sharing the demons I have grappled with, and how I managed to loosen myself from their grip, I can help others avoid them. It's taken me ten years to truly find my own mission within the wild west of the fitness world, and I am so grateful to have the opportunity to share it with you. As I hope you've gathered by now, this is not a prescriptive 'my way or the highway' kind of book. I want to change the way you think about exercise, not as punishing and painful but as exciting, challenging and invigorating.

Being able to move our bodies is a luxury that we

won't have for ever and I want to inspire you to enjoy every minute of it, not by telling you what to do, but by inspiring you to think about why, what, when and how you do it. This is the way I now approach fitness. I hope that in sharing what I've learned, I can guide you to the same happy place where I find myself now.

PART TWO
You

In the first section of this book, I laid bare all that went before me in terms of the mistakes I made and the things I learned along the way. But it wouldn't make sense to simply end the book there. My goal in writing this book is to not only show you the 'before' part of my journey but also to walk you step by step through the 'after', so I can help make sure that your journey is different from my own. I've learned so much over the last ten years, making mistakes along the way so you don't have to. If today is the day you're starting on your journey of finding strength, I want to ensure that you enjoy the process and see it as a commitment to yourself to start the journey with love and compassion for yourself and your body. After all, that's the most important foundation to build from.

It is also essential to see this as an opportunity to prioritize your health and wellbeing over how you might have previously tracked your progress, for example by aiming for a number on the scales or a dress size. Try and view today as the first day of a commitment to lasting, sustainable change rather than a diet that you follow for a few weeks, but give up after a short while because you end up feeling exhausted, losing momentum and not seeing changes happening quickly enough. Today is your day to engage with some positive new habits, to find a love for moving your body in a way you genuinely enjoy and to see the difference in yourself – both physically and mentally – from doing so.

For a long time fitness consumed me; it was all or nothing, and I had a punishing routine that I tried hard to keep up with, but in reality left me feeling flat. Coming away from this way of training has shown me that, while fitness is still incredibly important to me and something I enjoy hugely, it isn't my whole life. I want you to get to this place too. Where fitness is a happy addition to a fulfilling life; something that you do to make yourself feel good – not bad – about your body. I feel passionately about helping all women to achieve this. Understanding the WHY behind your training, separating fact from fiction and seeing how you can move your body in a way that you enjoy instead of it feeling like a chore or a punishment; there is, I believe, no better feeling.

This section of the book is broken down into four categories that I've developed as an easy guide for you to dip in and out of when you're looking for support on your exercise journey. It explores my four foundations of fitness: the WHY, the WHAT, the HOW and the WHEN. I really wanted to make this section as simple as possible; so often fitness professionals can overcomplicate things and spin you into a state of confusion. That's the opposite of what I want to do. I want to explain my ethos, clearly and thoroughly, so that when you close the final page of this book you've got a good understanding of everything you want to do for your own fitness journey. By understanding these elements, I hope you will be empowered with the knowledge to carve your own path to learn what works for you, so you can feel more in tune with your body and develop a lasting, loving relationship with it that isn't built on restriction or punishment.

It's important to say that this section isn't solely about training with weights and other equipment in the gym. While strength training is something I am passionate about and is how I personally choose to move my body, it is just one kind of exercise; there are quite literally hundreds of other brilliant choices. You might read this and decide strength training is for you, or you might not, and both decisions are okay. Either way, I will walk you through every part of this progressive new approach to your WHY, your WHAT, your WHEN and your HOW, which I can guarantee will help you to rebuild and realign every aspect of your approach to wellbeing.

As I mentioned in Part 1, I've written books before. I always got a sense back then that everyone in the publishing team wanted a 'big sell', and a guarantee of what the person reading the book is going to get from picking it up. I'm so grateful that when it came to writing this book, I wasn't pushed in that way. Of course, I hope that this book is a transformation of sorts for you, but not in the way that we are usually sold in the fitness industry, with the classic before and after photos to lure you in. I'm not expecting you to have an overnight epiphany. This book is about helping you to see the benefit of really wiping the slate clean and starting again with the objective of building habits for the long term, habits that will benefit your health, your sanity and your wellbeing. It's time to step off the dieting merry-go-round and really promise yourself change for good.

I want you to sail through this process not feeling pressured or obligated, but with a genuine desire to reconnect with the authentic you that existed before life told you that you needed to look a different way. Or before you used unhealthy habits to shrink yourself and saw that as a benchmark of your ideal body. I cannot stress enough that there is no point in looking 'the best you've ever looked' if you're not *feeling* your best or if it isn't sustainable in the long term.

A different approach to fitness

I have nearly a decade of professional personal training experience, working with all kinds of wonderful clients, so this feels like a natural place to start. I've spent the last eight years working hard both on the gym floor and online. Despite starting out on a shaky footing, I have made it my mission to really develop my skills to become the experienced trainer I am today. I've had such a vast array of clients with varying needs, abilities and goals and this has really helped me to develop not only my confidence as a coach but also my understanding of how to get someone from A to B effectively and sustainably. When I first started training clients, it was almost assumed that every client who came to you would have a weight-loss goal. My whole personal training qualification was set up to teach me how to help people lose weight, and every part of the industry was geared towards preying on vulnerable people by shaming them into an often overbearing exercise regime. There was little talk about recovery or rest days. In fact, when writing this book I flicked back through my old workbooks from a personal training course I took and was shocked at how much the education I was being given was centred around weight transformations. It was almost assumed that that would be the only type of client personal trainers would be working with.

While I've worked with a variety of methods, my passion and expertise now lie predominantly within strength training, more specifically helping women to build lean muscle and get physically stronger. As I made the shift to coaching clients away from fat loss and towards more positive and tangible exercise outcomes, a personal trainer I worked with criticized me heavily online. The conversation went like this:

Them: ***'You say you're not a weight-focused trainer. What if you get someone that needs that? Would they not be able to train with you?***

Me: ***'What I offer is a safe place to exercise for other benefits beyond fat loss. I have absolutely had cases where clients***

have come to me to lose weight, but I haven't felt the need to weigh them to tell them that. We work on introducing healthy habits, a consistent exercise routine, etc. For most women, the scales are a triggering place and if I can help them reach their goals, whatever they may be, without having to put them on the sad step, then I'm doing a good job.'

Them: '*Ok cool, all I'm saying is, there are people who need the scales, and to be weighed. If as a personal trainer you cannot do that, then you are failing those people. Forcing your beliefs on to them.'*

By this point, I was getting really annoyed.

Me: '*And that's what makes the world go round. I won't be everyone's cup of tea, no. But for some people I really am.'*

And here's the best line in his response: '*I pride myself on being a chameleon and adapting to my clients' needs. Not deciding what's best for them myself and thinking I know best just because "women power" and stuff.'*

I rest my case.

You see, it was hard at the beginning to buck the trend. To go against the grain of what had always been the heart of the fitness industry. To do something different riled some people immensely. How dare I put my clients' well-being first and get them to the same end point without the need to shame them or create a potentially lifelong poor relationship with both their body and with exercise?

Thankfully, I had the confidence to continue with my pursuit of doing what I believed was best for my clients and those who followed me. I've always been deeply conscious of the responsibility that comes from having a large platform. As I navigated my own course and turned my back on weighing myself, and exercising solely to lose weight, I just knew that there would be those who followed me who totally agreed with my approach.

As you've read in Part 1 of this book, when I was growing up my only experience of exercise outside of school sports was seeing my mum punish herself with exercise she didn't enjoy in order to lose weight. People have been doing this for years and it's for the most part because this is how exercise has been sold to us. Exercise, and how it's been packaged up to us by the fitness industry, has so often been centred around how we look. You only have to recall certain high street gyms who roll out the same toxic rhetoric each January, guilt-shaming people into joining the gym because they might have eaten a little more over the Christmas period. And look, I'm not here to judge you if that is your motivation, but I want to encourage you to think bigger and beyond that too. It's not fundamentally wrong to have aesthetic goals (in fact it is totally normal and understandable!) but it's my view that they will only see you so far. They are just one piece of the puzzle; what I want is for you to think about the whole picture, for the long rather than the short term, and to consider more than just how you look, and instead focus on the many other positive factors that could and should motivate you on your health journey. If that sounds like something that you'd like to try, then you're in the right place.

The school sports conundrum

Before we move on, I think it's important to reflect on our early experiences with formal exercise as these often shape how we feel as we get older. For many of us, this begins at school, with PE lessons we have to do while gaining an education. Some of you may have had a wholly positive experience with sport at school but for many it can be the start of a reluctant and depressing relationship with exercise.

I personally never excelled at PE or found it enjoyable; the uniforms were exposing and it often felt like a chore. More than anything, I was just grateful every time it was over. At secondary school I'd do whatever I could to avoid sports classes, and I know I wasn't the only one. Many of my friends – as well as women I've worked with – say they had the exact same experience. And I really believe that if we get off on the wrong foot with exercise, it can have a lasting impact.

It isn't just anecdotal evidence that shows this. Stats from Women in Sport UK show us the clear inequality between boys and girls when it comes to sports at school. In 2022, girls were significantly less active than boys, with a gap of 213,000 (47 per cent of boys were active compared to 43 per cent of girls). Girls' participation in team sports was also much lower than boys', at only 41 per cent compared to 63 per cent. A further important barrier to entry was shown to be ethnicity, with only 28 per cent of Black British girls being active at school, which was down a huge 8 per cent from the previous year.

And when it comes to the enjoyment of exercise – a crucial pillar for long-term success – just over a third of girls (34 per cent) in Years 9 to 11 say they enjoy taking part in sports and exercise compared to more than half of boys (55 per cent).

Surely this demonstrates that our first exposure to movement is crucial and yet, when you consider all of this, it becomes clear that women (and particularly young women and those of colour) struggle with connecting to exercise from an early age. If (like me!) you weren't one of the sporty kids, you may have felt put off from the whole experience and avoided engaging with it again.

There are, of course, other reasons why girls often disengage from sports. Many feel uncomfortable exercising during their period, for instance, or uninspired by the narrow selection of options they might have to choose from: at my sixth form, for example, girls had to play netball, whereas the boys had five or six sports to choose from. Or how there have been fewer female sporting role models because women's sport has consistently received less funding than men's. Ultimately, it's clear that so many women don't pursue exercise at school or beyond because they disengage from it early on in their life, and often the overriding messaging is clear: 'If you're good, you're good and if you're not, don't bother.' We have to do better.

I believe our experience of sport at school really shapes the narratives we tell ourselves about exercise, even after we've left the education system. It's why so many of us only re-engage with exercise when we feel we have to, namely because we want to change our physical appearance. For so many of us, it's only sold to us in two rigid boxes – our experience at school, which often scars and scares us, and our experience as adults, which we start again begrudgingly because we want to lose weight.

Remember that iconic scene in *Bridget Jones's Diary* where she suddenly decides that a physical transformation (despite her healthy figure!) is necessary to overcome her heartbreak? We see Bridget slogging it out on a cross-trainer, which hammers home the unhelpful message that exercise is only to be picked up when we want to change how we look, and to improve our desirability to the opposite sex. Or the countless other shows where women lose weight and have a 'glow up' and are suddenly seen as attractive. We're drip-fed messages like this from such a young age, and yet the idea that exercise is only worth it if we want to be desired more is incredibly reductive and damaging – to us, our relationship with exercise and the romantic relationships we pursue.

Wouldn't it be amazing if, from a young age, we really understood how important movement was for our overall wellbeing? Not just our physical health, but for our mood, cognitive function, sleep and stress levels.

Wouldn't it be brilliant if we learned about the benefits of donning our PE kit and heading outside on a cold day rather than it seeming like nothing more than an obligatory and often miserable experience? When we frame exercise in a positive way, both with the language we use and the narrative we tell, it becomes so much easier to make it far more inclusive and get everyone engaged. But sadly, so many of us aren't afforded that pleasure, so we cycle along a rough pathway that so frequently includes losing interest in school sports, and then later on becoming locked in a punishing cycle where we exercise because we want to lose weight, without ever finding the joy of how movement can be a wonderful and positive addition to life.

I wish my PE teachers had really schooled us on how health and fitness is nothing to do with how you look. Looking a certain way doesn't automatically make you 'healthy' – I definitely learned that the hard way. Once I realized this crucial point and instead started focusing on how my body felt and functioned, I could listen to my body more intuitively, embrace it and nurture it, and really create a solid foundation for feeling good in the long term. And I want that same outcome for you.

The four foundations

I'd like to lay out my four foundations of fitness and see how we can make each one work for you. Regardless of where you are on your journey, these are the principles I want you to keep coming back to, revisiting them whenever you feel like you aren't enjoying your routine as much, or when you want to shift your focus. The best thing about these foundations is that they are all jumping-off points for you to make your own. They aren't instructions, but questions for you to answer, and your answers may well change as you move through life.

I don't believe in setting rigid rules, and this isn't a prescriptive programme you have to stick to day in day out. Instead, this is something that should evolve alongside you as you grow and change over the weeks, months and years ahead. When it comes to health and fitness, we must remember that we are all so different. There is no 'one-size-fits-all' approach. We need to let go of comparison and trying to keep up with what others are doing and become more attuned to our own bodies and minds.

As you work through my four foundations of fitness, I want you to learn to prioritize what makes you *feel* good rather than what you think makes you *look* good. That is the key. Trial and error will be your best friend as you discover what works for you, what fits with your lifestyle, what puts a smile on your face and makes you feel nourished, connected, challenged and – ultimately – strong.

I have been through a few turbulent years of struggling to find a happy place with my body and with exercise, but I have finally discovered what gives me strength, mentally and physically. I want nothing more than for you to find that in these pages too. So, let's now embark on this exciting new journey. Take a deep breath and together, let's throw out the old and bring in the new.

5. Why

Before we start digging deeper into finding your own personal WHY, let's think about why it's so important that we move. Exercise is a fundamental part of who we are as humans. We are designed to move and run and jump, and yet our lifestyles are increasingly sedentary, which isn't good for our bodies or our health.

The physical benefits of exercise are vast. They include (and this isn't a totally exhaustive list): lower mortality risk, increased mobility and flexibility, increased bone density and improved proprioception and balance. I truly believe that when it comes to preventative measures to stave off almost all the things we can fear falling ill with, exercise should be up there as one of the most prescribed treatments for its benefits. According to the NHS in the UK, if you're doing the recommended 150 minutes of exercise each week, on average you should experience 35 per cent less risk of heart disease and stroke, 20 per cent less risk of developing breast cancer and 50 per cent less risk of colon cancer. While these are just a handful of statistics, they clearly demonstrate how critical regular movement can be to achieving positive health outcomes and increased longevity.

The mental benefits of exercise are also extensive. Most of us will know the feeling at the end of a workout when you get that rush of endorphins and a boost of happiness. Beyond that, regular movement is known to decrease the risk of depression by 30 per cent. It also improves sleep quality, memory, body image and cognitive function, helps to manage anxiety, relieve stress, provide social connections and so much more.

While I do think it's important to understand why exercise is so good for us, I don't believe that this information is particularly groundbreaking or new for you, and it's important to understand that it is rarely this knowledge that motivates us to exercise. I don't know many people who rush to the gym simply to 'improve their bone density'; I certainly don't. But it's nonetheless essential to appreciate the context of why a long-term sustainable exercise routine is so important.

It's also worth adding to this that positive health behaviours breed positive health behaviours. When you start to exercise from a positive place and you feel the compounding effects of regular exercise on your mood, sleep, stress and overall wellbeing, you will likely find yourself wanting to continue doing what you're doing. And this feeling of wellbeing can seep into other behaviours across your life too, such as your food choices and your body image. So while it might not be the driving factor, understanding the importance of regular movement is a valuable piece of the puzzle.

Find the fun

One of the biggest learnings that I want you to take from this book is understanding the connection between enjoying your chosen form of movement and your likelihood of continuing to practise it in the long term. We know that many gyms report a high dropout rate in the 3–6-month period after joining, and this is just one example of what can often happen with people's relationship to exercise. We start, we don't enjoy it, we lose interest and then we give it up.

This isn't a bad thing, it's totally understandable. Nobody wants to do something regularly that they don't enjoy. But it should be clear that if you do enjoy however you choose to move your body, you will be far more likely to stick to that way of moving.

Before we get into anything else, I want you to really think about what you enjoy when it comes to how you move. Maybe it's dancing round your kitchen with your favourite playlist on. Perhaps it's the community and feel-good vibes of CrossFit. Or maybe it's taking yourself to your local pool and doing some slow and steady laps. I'm not here to dictate how you should move; in fact, quite the opposite. I want you to explore your relationship with exercise, and really identify what brings you joy and makes you feel great.

As much as I love all types of movement, as a personal trainer who specializes in strength training, I do believe this to be an important component of a balanced approach to fitness, especially for women. This doesn't have to mean you need to sign up to a gym though. Home workouts, Pilates, calisthenics and body-weight workouts all count as resistance training, so perhaps it's about reframing what strength training looks like to you and finding something that you genuinely enjoy and fits into your lifestyle.

Enjoyment is everything. I'd like nothing more than to hear from someone who has read this book and ditched the punishment of exercise they didn't like, and has instead chosen to listen to their body and explore movement they do enjoy. So this is your chance to rip up what you 'think' you should be doing because it 'burns the most calories' (we will come to this later) and instead allow yourself to really find some feel-good movement.

Motivation

For us to exercise consistently, we need the motivation to get moving. This underpins every conscious action we take when it comes to working on our health and wellbeing. We need to feel motivated to get out of our warm cosy beds and put on our leggings to work out. We definitely need motivation when it's minus 3 degrees outside but we've committed to going for a run. For many, motivation can be the most difficult thing to come by, like there is a disconnect between knowing we need to move because it's good for us, and actually having the motivation to do it.

I firmly believe that figuring out what you enjoy is the best place to start when it comes to finding your motivation to move and regularly reminding yourself of this is key to moving forward with your goals. If you hate running but decide to start doing it, it's unlikely you're going to stick to it in the long term, which will only make you feel worse about yourself because you'll think you've failed. The enjoyment must be there.

While enjoyment is a crucial part of my ethos and approach to exercise, I'm under no illusion that it's easy to come by the first time you try something. The first time I tried weight training I was extremely self-conscious; it took a lot of energy to convince myself to go back and do it again. I just felt this pressure to get it first time. If you're anything like me, there is a certain amount of ego involved when it comes to trying new things, and I admit that I simply don't enjoy stuff as much when I'm not good at it. Strength training was a real lesson for me in learning to drop my ego and be a beginner again, and I encourage you to do the same. See the challenge of starting something new and enjoy the journey of getting better. We all have to start somewhere and we all have to be a beginner once. That said, it's understandable that for a lot of us, if we're not instantly 'good' at something, we don't feel a burning urge to do it again. So most of us do need other tricks in our toolkit to help us lock in some much-needed motivation.

Understanding the psychology of motivation has really helped me to form a better approach to building and sustaining it in the long term, and there are two categories of motivation that we need to draw upon to help us stick to our chosen form of movement in the long term: intrinsic and extrinsic motivation. This draws on the idea that rather than relying on one thing to motivate us, such as the enjoyment of exercise, we need multiple tools in our hypothetical motivation toolkit to get us exercising consistently.

Extrinsic motivation is when we engage in an activity because we want to earn some kind of reward. This means you will engage in a behaviour because you expect to get something from it. This could look like participating in a sport to win awards or going for a run with a group so you can make new friends while you exercise. This is where fitness events or challenges can be brilliant. They provide us with a focus, but also offer the possibility of a reward at the end. For me, events aren't my favourite way to stay motivated as I find the pressure of them too much. When it comes to extrinsic motivation within my own training environment, this is where tracking my sessions and monitoring my progress have been crucial in ensuring I train regularly. There really is no better feeling than being able to have tangible proof that I'm getting consistently stronger from the hard work I'm putting in at the gym. So don't worry if signing up to an event isn't for you either. There are many ways in which you can engineer tangible outcomes from your training.

Intrinsic motivation differs in that it comes from

within and is when you engage in a behaviour because of how it makes you feel. While extrinsic motivators can come and go across your lifetime, intrinsic motivators remain relatively consistent, and it's about dialling into them to make them work for you in the long term. When I think about my own intrinsic motivators, I often remind myself of the benefits of exercise that go beyond how I look. For example, I focus on how it eases my stress and clears my mind, how it can improve my body image, how it helps me to feel more focused and gives me a sense of accomplishment every time I finish a session. It is these cues that I will remind myself of when I need an extra nudge to go to the gym.

The important thing to remember is that there is no right or wrong when it comes to what motivates you to move. But have a think about your WHYs and then focus in on some tangible motivators that will help you to keep consistent with your training. This will go a long way to helping you have an enduring, positive relationship with exercise.

I find that setting myself specific training goals helps me to focus on really enjoying my training rather than simply watching the 'calorie burn' accrue on my fitness tracker and only being satisfied with my workout when I'd hit a certain number. Setting yourself specific goals within your chosen form of training can be a brilliant way to keep yourself motivated. They don't have to be huge challenges like running a marathon or squatting 100kg; they can be as simple as improving how you do a given exercise or going for a little longer than last time when you head out for your weekly run. Having some focus within your training that isn't just wanting to change your outer appearance can be a really positive way to reframe your relationship with exercise. In my experience working as a personal trainer, the clients who got the most from their training were the ones who committed to working on specific goals such as doing a pull-up or hitting a deadlift PB, no matter how big or small.

That said, clients rarely come to me with the initial motivation to work on a specific training goal. For example, almost every client would come to me wanting to change their body composition in some way. I never tell people that what they want to achieve is wrong because every goal is valid, but as I explained at the start of this section, as much as I listened and took on their goals, I also worked with them to try and place more of a focus on how their body moved and functioned rather than what they looked like. I would concentrate on establishing a less rigid, more fun and explorative workout on the gym floor that was all about what their body could do; following this, more often than not they would revise their whole approach. That simple switch would be game-changing.

Goals in training

I've learned some really useful tips over the years when it comes to goal setting. While I appreciate that having goals can sometimes be a distraction or a hindrance, I do believe that for the majority of people they provide a lifeline, allowing you to focus on something far more rewarding than the number on the scales.

If you're struggling to quantify what your specific goal or goals might be, there is a popular technique used in the fitness industry (and elsewhere) to help you to define what you want to achieve. It's called the SMART approach and it's useful when you need some clearer understanding of your goals and how you can realistically get yourself there.

SPECIFIC I always say to my clients that random training gets you random results. The more specific you are with what you want to achieve, the more you will be able to focus on what you need to do to get there. If you want to achieve a full push-up, for example, you need to be doing push-ups within your training as well as some upper body strength work each week.

MEASURABLE This is where weight training can be so brilliant. If you're tracking your weights each week, it's very easy to have a tangible measure of progression. While it's important to remember that progress is not always linear, having a proper log of each session will help you to see clear trends of strength progression, even if the line doesn't go straight upwards.

ACHIEVABLE While it's great to have big ambitions when it comes to your training, goals that are too far out of our reach can actually have a negative impact on our motivation to train, as they feel too unachievable.

Having goals that are ambitious *and* achievable is the sweet spot. So make sure you choose something that feels doable for you and where you're at with your training.

RELEVANT When you're setting training goals it's essential that you make them relevant to you. Rather than trying to copy someone on Instagram or trying to change your body to look like someone else's, your goals should be *by* you and *for* you – period. When you're deciding what you want to work towards, try and block out other people's influences and hone in on what's important to you and where you're at.

TIMELY Having a time frame on your goals can be really helpful to motivate you. If you have a never-ending period of working towards something, there is no immediacy to your actions. And while I don't believe in quick fixes, setting a realistic target date for your goals can help to provide the focus you need.

It's important to note here that just as any progress is rarely linear, your journey to your goals can be non-linear too. It rarely happens that you go from A to B in one straight line, and in some ways this is part of the 'fun' of the journey. So please don't let a squiggly line from your start to your end goal put you off or make you think you aren't doing great. It's also okay to be quite fluid with a goal. I've certainly made the mistake of being so tied to a goal that it started to rule me, so allow yourself to be flexible. If you feel a target isn't helping or contributing to your training, perhaps try focusing on smaller and simpler goals instead, like sticking to something for a week or a month or having a daily step count target. Opt for things that are not going to affect your mood or motivation negatively instead. I admit it's a balancing act, and one that might take a while to adjust to, but it will be worth it in the long term.

Once you've made clear what some of your goals might be and what they look like, it can be helpful to then break them down into two categories: macro and micro goals. Macro goals will be your big overarching goals. This could be, for example, wanting to deadlift your own body weight, to run 5km in a specific time or to achieve your first pull-up. It's the stuff that takes a little longer to get to, but with consistency and hard work can be achieved. In contrast to this, micro goals are the stuff you do every day, or every week. These are smaller, easily achieved things to tick off your list. Mine tend to be things like hitting a step count every day, drinking a certain amount of water and hitting a certain number of gym sessions each week. They shouldn't be hard to maintain, but they're mini targets that can keep you focused on the day-to-day stuff while you work towards your macro goal.

A big caveat here is that while I do believe having goals is important, I've also gone through periods of my own training where I've put them on pause and simply exercised for enjoyment and fun, with less of a focus on achieving anything and more of a focus on simply moving my body because it feels good. Some of us will thrive on being constantly goal-orientated, and some of us will go through cycles with goals where we give ourselves a little breather too.

It's okay to experience periods where you just don't have goals because you're simply enjoying moving when you can, and that's enough. This is particularly important to remember if you're going through a stressful or busy time, when goals can be an added pressure because you've already got enough on your to-do list. So please remember that while goals can be great, I am also the first person to encourage you to drop or pause them if they're not serving the purpose they're designed to.

Moving through life

Your WHY can change too. It doesn't have to be something that you're chained to for your entire life. It will naturally grow and evolve as you do, but really thinking about why you want to exercise can be the perfect first task to start your own healing process.

In my twenties I did far too many heavy gym sessions per week with little respect for recovery or mobility, and there was only so long that my body could sustain that. As we age, our bodies still need to move, but rest and recovery becoming increasingly important. My approach has thankfully evolved to incorporate quality over quantity in my gym sessions, as well as mobility on my rest days. This has meant that my training has in fact got better as a result, as my body is getting adequate rest (and I'm also fuelling the training I am doing properly too). Learning to adapt your training to where you are in your life can feel like a hard thing to get your head around when coming from a background of thinking that 'surely the more exercise, the better', but it can make all the difference to your ability to continue exercise through life consistently. No one expects you to be doing the same amount or type of exercise at eighty that you did at eighteen. Making adaptations to scale your workouts to where you're at is key.

This is particularly important for women. We know that our bodies can have big hormonal shifts across our lifetime, and while exercising will always be important, why you exercise might heavily depend on where you find yourself in life. If you're post-natal, for example, your approach to training will be very different to someone going through perimenopause or having menopause symptoms, and very different again from someone in their early twenties who might be able to tolerate a higher training threshold. My whole approach to exercise now takes into account that it's vitally important to be conscious of what serves you at each point of your life, and it's absolutely okay if your priorities and goals within exercise shift continuously as you do.

The calorie burn myth

My final note in this chapter is the much-discussed subject of calorie burn. The amount of energy that you expend during exercise is something that with the rise of fitness trackers has meant almost all of us now have access to some kind of metric that tells us what we've 'burned' during a workout. This is why a lot of us will opt for high-intensity workouts or will stay in the gym or on a treadmill for longer than we want to; because a device on our wrist is telling us we've not done enough to equate to a 'good workout'. It makes for a relationship with exercise that becomes more focused on data rather than enjoyment, and often means people become far less intuitive with their workouts. This is highly problematic when it comes to creating a positive relationship with exercise for a few reasons.

The first is that nearly all the most commonly worn fitness trackers can be wildly inaccurate. A recent evaluation conducted at the Stanford University School of Medicine examined seven different fitness trackers. In their findings, NONE of these devices measured energy expenditure accurately, with even the most accurate device being off by an average of 27 per cent and the least accurate by 93 per cent. So while it might feel as though by wearing a fitness tracker you're more in control of your energy output, the reality is that the number you're being shown is very often far from what you've actually expended.

The second reason is that it can create a dynamic in your workouts whereby you're solely working out to see the numbers clock up on your wrist rather than being more intuitive and in tune with your body during your session. I know there were times in my disordered eating and overexercising phase when I would literally force myself to carry on training, even when my workout should have finished, to make sure I got to '300 calories' or '400 calories'. It was such a toxic mindset and it meant that I was only satisfied when I was able to work hard enough to hit those targets.

It's important to say that this doesn't mean that I'm against fitness trackers. They can be a helpful addition to some people's lives (remember the MEASURABLE in the SMART goals mentioned above?), but I do think that it's particularly important to be in control of your relationship with your tracker rather than it being in control of you. If you find yourself opting for the higher calorie burn workouts, or constantly monitoring your wrist during exercise to see how much energy you're expending, perhaps try going without your fitness tracker for a while. And when it comes to finding your WHY, please don't let it be calories that dictate your progress. Our ways of measuring them are often inaccurate, so obsessing over them is not going to be effective in achieving weight loss (more on this later) and it's going to keep you locked in a cycle of only feeling you've done a 'good enough' workout when the numbers tell you so rather than that belief coming from you.

You need to remind yourself that a watch cannot gauge how you're feeling mentally or physically. It's simply a device used to read your heart rate and tell you roughly how many steps you've done. So don't give it more power than it deserves. Only you know what you're experiencing, so try the process of weaning yourself off it and see if it makes a difference.

6. What

Once you understand WHY you want to move, it will hopefully become easier to work out WHAT ways of moving your body might be best for you. Whether it's running because you work at home and want to get outside more, or weight training to build your strength to feel more capable and confident – this section is all about helping you find your WHAT.

While there is no single right way to exercise because, as we know, that will look different for all of us, finding your WHAT is all about making exercise sustainable. The crucial aspect is that it should be something you're able to stick to in the long term. There's no point in taking up swimming if the nearest pool is 30 minutes away and you never end up going, or in putting yourself through spinning classes simply because everyone else is doing it, even though you hate every minute.

I think one of the reasons it can be challenging to create a lasting relationship with our WHAT is that often once we find something we genuinely enjoy, we then come out of the blocks fast, chasing results and wanting them quickly. It's understandable, right? You enjoy moving your body, it makes you feel good and you want results. So more = better. But often this level of intensity can be unsustainable and there's a good chance you will literally run out of puff and lose interest or feel deflated that you can't sustain that amount of training for a prolonged period of time.

While I'd hope that by now you've worked to discover your WHY and that you appreciate the value of going beyond aesthetics, it is true that this undoubtedly influences many of our choices when it comes to our WHAT. If I had a pound for every time someone messaged me with, 'What's the best exercise I can do to get in shape FAST?' I'd be laughing all the way to the bank. And although I empathize with this approach, there are many myths when it comes to exercise that tend to push people towards certain things and away from others. For example:

- Cardio is good for fat loss.
- Strength training makes you bulky.
- Yoga isn't a hard enough workout.
- Pilates is only for women.

I could go on! These are all inaccurate statements that a lot of us are fooled by; unfortunately, they are also reasons why people continue to punish themselves with exercise that they might not enjoy.

There are quite literally hundreds of ways to move your body that will benefit your health in both the short and long term, from hiking and swimming to boxing and ballet. Finding a way of moving that you enjoy and that fits with your WHY at this moment in time is the number one foundation on which to build your exercise journey. That means that you might have to try out a few things before you settle on something that works for you, but I guarantee you that there is a type of exercise that works for all of us.

All movement matters

When it comes to WHAT movement we should be doing, there is so much more going on than meets the eye. When we limit our view of exercise to extreme spin classes or bootcamps, it distracts us from all the small things we do each day that add up to more daily movement. From a physiological perspective, there are two types of energy expenditure that we typically look at in relation to our long-term health and wellbeing: our EAT (exercise activity thermogenesis) and NEAT (non-exercise activity thermogenesis). To make things very simple, we want to be both EATing and NEATing and I'll explain why.

EAT is the amount of energy you expend when doing structured exercise. Whether it's running, hiking, strength training or cycling, whatever exercise you do contributes to your overall energy expenditure each day.

NEAT is the amount of energy we expend during daily activities, not including sleeping, eating and exercising. It's things like playing with your kids, walking to work, doing the laundry, hoovering and even just standing. Every movement we make uses energy and while that expenditure can seem small, it can make a substantial difference as it accumulates over time.

Before I explain any more about this, it's important to put NEAT into an overall energy context, also known as our total daily energy expenditure, or TDEE. Our TDEE is broken down into different categories, as shown below.

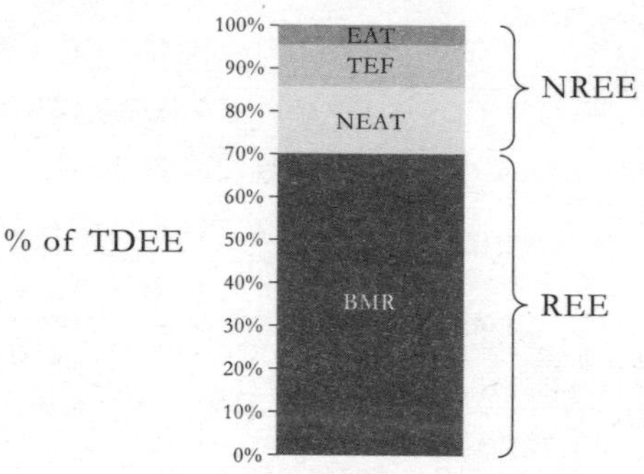

- REE is our resting energy expenditure. This constitutes around 60–75 per cent of our TDEE and includes our sleeping, basal and arousal metabolism. REE is the number of calories a body needs at rest to perform basic functions such as keeping the heart beating and the brain functioning.
- The rest of the energy used is classified as NREE, or non-resting energy expenditure. This is further broken down into different subcategories, including EAT and NEAT

(which we've already covered) and TEF, which stands for thermic effect of food.

- TEF constitutes around 10 per cent of our total TDEE and describes the energy that is required to operate our digestive processes and absorption and assimilation of food nutrients. The magnitude of TEF can vary depending on both the quantity and type of food eaten.

What this shows us is that, far from being crucial for burning calories, exercise activity thermogenesis (EAT) only makes up around 5 per cent of our TDEE, whereas non-exercise activity thermogenesis (NEAT) is the most variable component of our metabolism and can be anything from 15 to 20 per cent of TDEE.

The problem with relying on NEAT energy expenditure is that so many of us now find ourselves stuck behind a desk for eight hours a day, and the majority of our NEAT comes from minimal activity like grabbing a coffee or walking up the stairs. But if you incorporate more movement into your daily routine (see some practical tips on this on page 193), you can make a big difference to the amount of NEAT energy you accrue, which in turn improves your overall wellbeing.

Another issue with working out hard and focusing on a high calorie burn is that you will use up a lot of energy, which means you will start getting hungry. The body tries to maintain balance by altering two important hormones called ghrelin and leptin, which control satiety and hunger, so you may find yourself with a spike in appetite, which can lead to you overeating. In my time spent practising pretty disordered habits with food and exercise, the excessive hunger I experienced following a hard workout could indeed lead to all-out binges. Rather than addressing my overall energy balance and properly fuelling my training, I obsessed over each calorie and this instead led to me falling into the difficult binge–restrict cycle.

So NEAT can be used effectively in a more positive and sustainable approach to exercise; it has been shown to help manage these hormones over time, which can be helpful for long-term, sustainable health and wellbeing.

Another drawback of only ever thinking of training hard and eating less is that in response – sometimes without even realizing it – we naturally become more sedentary in order to retain energy. So while it might seem as though several hard workouts a week is proving your 'dedication', in actual fact an excessively high training volume could be making you move less overall, not more.

As we work towards changing the narrative around NEAT, it's important to understand that movement is also helpful for many other processes within our body, including our digestion and motility of food, our lymphatic system and our general mental health. So whatever your goal, movement outside of the gym is a brilliant thing to build into your new approach to exercise and is something that should be framed as good for your head and your heart, without obsessing over 'calories burned' or 'step count'.

How to increase your NEAT

There may already be moments during your day when you're thinking you might be able to squeeze in a cheeky walk, for instance, but if you're struggling for inspiration, consider whether any of the below might be possible for you:

- Getting off the bus/tube/train one stop earlier to walk the last part of your journey.
- Using the stairs instead of taking the lift.
- Standing instead of sitting at your desk, or replacing your chair with a stability ball.
- Getting outside during your lunch break for a walk.
- Finding small ways to move when seated, such as gentle stretches.
- Setting a reminder to stand up at least once an hour to move.

We have become so obsessed with training hard (and trying to change our bodies) that the humble walk has been shunned by many. In fact, walking every day is one of the best things you can do for your overall health *and* it's both sustainable and enjoyable (well, when it's not raining). It's also joint-friendly and is something you will hopefully be able to do for the rest of your life, plus it's the least likely form of activity to spike your hunger.

What type of exercise is best?

This book is called *Give Me Strength*, partly because I want to inspire you to become physically and mentally stronger, but also because on a more basic level, I am passionate about helping women to increase their strength through weight training. My dream is for all women to try weight training and love it as much as I do, but I realize that for some people it just doesn't work, and that's okay. So, let's explore how you can find the way of training that works best for you.

I am asked so often what the best type of exercise is, mostly by those who want to lose weight and want the quickest solution. But the simple answer is that the best form of exercise you can do is the one you can stick to consistently in the long term. Say that again out loud, because it's something we often forget!

This said, there *are* some fundamentals to grasp when it comes to movement and our health. While all movement, regardless of its form, is going to be good for you, the wide variety of exercise available to us can be broken down into different subcategories, and it can be helpful to understand the pros and cons of each one, so you can see what might work best for you and your goals.

Aerobic/cardiovascular exercise

One of the biggest myths within the fitness industry is that cardio is the ultimate 'fat-burning' method. As I shared earlier, when I previously wanted to lose weight, my belief was that running on a treadmill to hit a certain calorie target was the only way. To be clear, cardiovascular training does indeed utilize energy. But guess what? So does everything you do, so please don't see cardio as the be-all and end-all. If you hate running, you don't have to run to be fit and healthy, I promise.

Cardiovascular training is important for all of us in some capacity, though. This is because training our heart and lungs to pump blood efficiently around the body is crucial for our overall wellbeing. Cardiovascular disease is the leading cause of death globally, and neglecting to include some small element of cardio training within your overall exercise routine can mean that you become less efficient with this process, less physically fit over time and – needless to say – more susceptible to cardiovascular disease.

So what is cardiovascular exercise? Running, cycling, swimming and brisk walking are all good examples. These forms of movement train the heart and lungs to be more efficient at transporting and utilizing oxygen and energy round the body.

When we do cardiovascular exercise, our body exerts energy and exercises our heart. There are different levels of intensity of cardiovascular exercise, which are often referred to as 'zones' and which I've set out below.

- **Zone 1** – 50–60 per cent of your heart's 'maximum output capacity' is everyday living and walking around.
- **Zone 2** – 60–70 per cent of your heart's capacity is going for a jog or a cycle, while still being able to hold a conversation.
- **Zone 3** – 70–80 per cent of your heart's capacity is going for a run or a cycle at a pace you can sustain but in conversation you can only give one- or two-word answers.
- **Zone 4** – 80–90 per cent of your heart's capacity is your lactic threshold zone, which is where you'll start to feel that unpleasant burn in your muscles as they fill with lactic acid. This type of training is typically done in short bouts like sprints.
- **Zone 5** – 90–100 per cent of your heart's capacity involves an all-out effort and is probably not sustainable for much more than 10–20 seconds.

Variety is key in any well-balanced fitness routine, so trying to span a range of heart rate zones is beneficial. A really good idea is to first build up a base level of fitness in the lower intensities, so that you can then establish tolerance and skill level. Once you're more confident, you can start to challenge yourself with more demanding heart rate zones.

I have recently started incorporating more running into my training for a few different reasons. Firstly, I'd neglected cardio for quite a while as I find it quite challenging, so I really lack motivation to stick to it (yes, I'm human and I lack motivation to exercise too!). Secondly, I wanted to generally feel a bit 'fitter' in my day-to-day life. I was finding myself more out of breath than I liked when walking up a few flights of stairs and in some gym exercises too. What's more, running is free and means getting outdoors, which gets me away from my phone and laptop; I thought it might even be something I came to enjoy in the long term. I used the zones listed above to make sure I wasn't overly exerting myself; I wanted to run for a prolonged period of time, so aiming for zone 2 was my goal. I'm pleased to say, having come at running this time around with a completely different, less pressured approach, where I simply focus on remaining in zone 2 (I track this using a fitness watch) regardless of distance or time, I am finally enjoying the process and am proud to have stuck to one run a week for the last five months.

However, if running isn't for you, that's totally okay too. There are many other ways you can incorporate cardiovascular training into your lifestyle including:

- **Fast uphill walking** – I love this as it involves a lower intensity on the joints, which means it's great if you're not a keen runner but still want to be hitting a similar intensity to jogging. Either find yourself a nice hilly route to walk regularly or jump on a treadmill and set the incline so that you're walking uphill and are roughly working in zone 2 (talking pace but still a little out of breath).
- **Swimming** – This is another option that is incredibly joint-friendly. Swimming can be such a brilliant way to include cardio in your training, and a lot of people enjoy the weightless feeling of being in the pool. Again, try and aim for zone 2 here, where you're feeling a little puffed but not totally exhausted, and gradually build up how many lengths you're able to do over time. I like to include swimming in my training around my menstrual cycle. When I'm due on my period or in the first few days of my period, I find the weightlessness of being in the pool really helpful.
- **Cycling** – What I love about cycling is that while also being more joint-friendly than running, it can be incredibly social too. My parents are long-time members of a cycling club and their weekends are filled with bike rides accompanied by coffee and cake along the way. If you have access to a bike, why not aim for

one ride a week, incorporating some hills into your route if you feel up to it? Aim for a time goal and slowly build up how long you're able to cycle for.

- **Dancing** – I mean, who doesn't love to dance? Coming from a dance background, I know first hand how brilliant dancing can be as a cardio workout, and if you're trying to foster a positive relationship with exercise, dancing as simply a fun way to move your body can be brilliant. Find out if there are any dance classes local to you where you feel confident to let go and enjoy the session, or alternatively, just switch on some music in your living room and set yourself a goal of having a boogie for 30 minutes. It's amazing how exhausting (and fun!) this can actually be.

Anaerobic exercise

If aerobic exercise is to do with the utilization of oxygen, anaerobic is the opposite. It is any activity that breaks down glucose for energy without using oxygen. Generally, these activities are of short length and with high intensity. Examples of anaerobic exercise include weightlifting, sprinting, cycling (in sprinting bouts) and any high-intensity interval training.

The idea is that a lot of energy is released within a small period of time, and your oxygen demand surpasses your body's oxygen supply. In order to cope, the body uses its anaerobic system, which relies on energy stores in the muscles. Anaerobic work used to be seen as the preserve of athletes training at a high level, but now that there are more and more 'everyday athletes' training in things like weightlifting, CrossFit and sprinting, many of us can and should reap the rewards of this type of training.

When you train at high levels of intensity, you increase your anaerobic threshold, which basically means you can then work harder for longer periods of time. Your longer workout sessions can improve as well. This is because through practising anaerobic exercise, you improve your VO2 max (the volume of oxygen your body uses when you are exercising as hard as you can), which means your body learns how to use more oxygen. It also leads to increased strength and stronger bones.

A good way to think about anaerobic exercise is that it's a good piece of the overall puzzle when it comes to fitness. A well-balanced training programme might aim to hit a bit of everything (aerobic, anaerobic and muscular endurance exercise) across the week. That doesn't mean you need to run a marathon, cycle 5km and deadlift your own body weight every seven days, but it gives you a good example of what a balanced programme might look like and what you'd perhaps want to include. The only caveat with anaerobic training is that sometimes the exercises or modalities required to hit this threshold can be on the more advanced end of the spectrum. Heavy deadlifts, fast sprints or sled pushes can all be slightly more demanding for the average gym-goer. If you're comfortable with these then that's great, but if you're not quite there yet, don't worry either.

Muscular endurance exercise

If aerobic training is consistently keeping an energy system going, and anaerobic is short, quick bouts of high-intensity energy, muscular endurance is the final key component. It involves the ability of a muscle or group of muscles to exert force consistently and repetitively for an extended period of time.

Muscle endurance is all about training your muscles to produce more force for longer. This could be within weight training on higher rep exercises, or in long-distance running or cycling, for example.

Within strength training, muscle endurance is about quantity of repetitions as much as quality, so it should be done with lighter weights. The greater your muscular endurance, the higher the number of repetitions you can complete. This type of training is most useful for targeting more isolated, smaller muscle groups such as your biceps or calves, rather than bigger muscle groups such as quads or pecs. Within my own training, I usually reserve this for things like high repetitions of bicep curls or cable kickbacks, where the total volume isn't going to affect my form as much.

I started this chapter by stating that I fundamentally believe there is no 'best' kind of exercise. It really is about whatever works best for you and what you enjoy. But I'm sure it won't come as a shock to hear that I am biased when it comes to weight training; it's one of my great passions and I truly believe it's something we should all be doing in some capacity.

During the healing journey with my relationship with exercise and my body, resistance training has been the thing that's really 'stuck' for me and seen me through some difficult times, whether that was after escaping my abusive relationship or when I finally acknowledged that training just to be smaller wasn't healthy for me. It's been something that has empowered me and made me feel more in touch with my body and myself than anything else. I sincerely believe that many of you would benefit from feeling the same strength and inspiration that I got – and continue to get – from weight training.

The first thing to explain here is what is meant by 'strength training', 'resistance training' or 'weight training'. I use these terms interchangeably because they all mean essentially the same thing. They are exercises that are designed to improve strength, power and/or endurance. Strength is the ability to produce and manage force. Force is calculated by mass (load) x acceleration (speed). So, really anything that applies a force to the body, or helps the body manage acceleration, can be called a strength training exercise.

Resistance training typically means using the body's resistance to complete exercises. Pilates could be seen as resistance training, as can exercises like push-ups, body weight squats and pull-ups. Weight training means incorporating an external load by adding things like dumbbells, barbells, kettlebells, and resistance bands to increase the demand placed upon the body. I use these two phrases interchangeably because during most weight training sessions, there will be elements of both. Also, the benefits discussed in this section apply to both resistance training and weight training, so you don't have to incorporate both if you'd rather do one over the other.

There is an overwhelming amount of research and evidence to support the benefits of weight training. And yet, for so long women have been put off from lifting heavy weights because men convinced us it was too masculine, and we were conned into believing it would make us 'bulky'. Because of this, I think it's important to have a bit of a deep dive into the reasons why resistance training can be so beneficial.

Firstly, it can make you physically stronger. Strength helps us undertake basic tasks such as carrying shopping and lifting heavy items, and minimizes the risk of injuries, fractures and breaks if we fall. I find it's actually quite a flex when I can lift things in day-to-day life that people don't expect me to be able to. People are often a bit shocked by how much weight a five-foot-one woman can lift, and I want to maintain that skill late into my life!

On a more scientific level, resistance training has profound beneficial effects on the musculoskeletal system, helping to prevent conditions such as osteoporosis, sarcopenia and lower back pain. This is particularly important for women, who are at a higher risk of suffering from osteoporosis than men, and who also have to contend with declining hormones in later life, which can exacerbate these conditions.

In addition, recent seminal research demonstrates that resistance training may positively affect risk factors such as insulin resistance, resting metabolic rate, glucose metabolism, blood pressure, body fat and gastrointestinal transit time, all of which are associated with poor health outcomes.

Admittedly, when it comes to lifting weights, the bar to entry is slightly higher and that can be a deterrent for some people. It's not quite as simple as lacing up your trainers and going for a run. But there are endless free resources online that can help even the most inexperienced beginner take up resistance training from home, so please rest assured it *is* for everyone.

Strength training has improved my own life immeasurably. I went from a girl who thought she wasn't good enough to take up any form of sport, to someone who can deadlift over 100kg and loves every second of it. It's empowered me in ways I could have only dreamed of previously. It's gifted me confidence, taught me so much and remained a part of my life consistently every week for the last eight years. So, as I said before, while I would never insist on it, I would love you to give it a go and discover the immensely positive differences it could make to your life too.

There's no rush!

I hope that I have clearly laid out the different types of exercise so you can have a better idea of WHAT your own approach to working out might look like.

There are so many ways to move your body and they all have their own benefits. Once you've worked out your WHY, your WHAT can be very flexible. For example, you might find that during the summer months you want to make the most of being outside when the weather is nice. That could translate as 2–3 runs per week, with one day set aside for resistance training. Then, in the winter months, you might want to avoid the bad weather by going to the gym to do three resistance training workouts, along with one indoor rowing session or swim.

The reality is that your WHAT can be as fluid as you want it to be as you move through life. Check in with yourself regularly to see what you feel will serve you best.

7. How

We've now covered the WHY and the WHAT in terms of your pathway to embracing movement in a positive, healthy and sustainable way, and this section is the next important piece of the puzzle. It is the putting together of all you've learned so far so you can begin your very own journey. The HOW is all about understanding what approach to exercise is right for you. We are all unique and so rather than setting specific routines or workouts for absolutely everyone reading this book, I've created a toolkit that will help you to be more autonomous with what you do and give you the ability to make decisions for yourself.

The first half of this chapter is general advice, which applies to everyone, whatever kind of exercise you've decided is right for you. The second half is practical advice relating to my personal favourite form of exercise (and you won't be surprised to hear that that's . . . weight training!). For those who aren't interested in working with weights, that is of course absolutely fine; just read the first part of this chapter and then skip to the next section, which is all about finding your WHEN.

How should I approach exercise?

This is something I get asked about a lot and so I often speak about it on my Instagram. I think this question highlights where we often go wrong with our approach to fitness. As I've already said, there is no one-size-fits-all approach and the question of what constitutes a 'good' workout is a very complex one to answer. Someone who runs marathons is clearly fit, but perhaps doesn't enjoy weight training, whereas someone who is exceptionally strong in the gym might loathe the idea of a long-distance race. Yet they're both clearly in good physical condition. What I want to stress is that there is no such thing as a universally 'good' workout; it's all about what works for you as an individual. On some days a good workout for me is a 60-minute weights session; on another it's a 30-minute brisk walk. Believing the myth that only a certain number of calories burned, or a certain amount of sweat, or a certain length of time qualifies as a 'good' workout is likely setting you up to have a problematic relationship with exercise, one that doesn't allow for the flexibility needed to establish long-term habits. I'd love you to have a relationship with exercise whereby you can really push yourself on some days, but also know when to pull back on others. It's essential that *you* decide what is 'enough' rather than having an arbitrary calorie target or time frame in mind.

If you focus on quantity over quality with your

workouts, you may find yourself falling into a state of fatigue, burnout and lack of motivation because you're likely constantly overriding your ability to listen to what your body really needs. When I describe what constitutes a good workout (within whatever activity you're doing), I usually break it down into the following questions, which you can continue to ask yourself as you progress on your exercise journey:

1. Are you getting better at the exercises or activities you're doing? This could be running a little further each time you head out for a run, or increasing the load you are working with in a deadlift. While progress in exercise can be non-linear, having a tangible measure of how you're improving can be brilliant feedback to show that you're moving in the right direction.
2. Is the quality of your movement getting better in the exercises you're doing? This could look like improving your skill-based exercises, like a push-up, for example. Each time you visit the exercise, is it feeling a little easier and are you feeling more confident within your body?
3. Do you feel like you're improving your overall fitness? This may be harder to see over the course of each individual session, but over time you might find that with consistency, your ability to do more for longer has improved. For example, you might be able to do three rounds

of sled pushes during your first few workouts, but a few months later, you find you're able to do five.

4. Are you feeling energized at the end of each session, or just exhausted? While tiredness after a hard workout is totally normal, you shouldn't be feeling as though you need to go and lie down. In fact, more often than not, exercise should *give* you energy rather than take it away. If you're finishing workouts and feeling totally wiped, you might want to readdress how much training you're doing and consider scaling it back a bit.
5. Are you having 'normal' hunger responses to your training? We know that as we increase our energy expenditure, our body responds by making us hungry so that we take in more food. With a balanced exercise routine, these hunger responses shouldn't be too much beyond what you would 'normally' eat. If, however, you're finding that you are extremely hungry post-workout and are needing to eat a lot to feel replenished, this might be a sign you're doing too much. (This advice doesn't apply to endurance-style training, which does require a big uptake of energy both before and after.)

Learning to ask yourself these questions can be a useful, more intuitive way of knowing if the exercise you're doing is right for you. It allows for a more personalized response and should help you see what a 'good' amount of training is for you.

Achieving progress

Now that we've discussed what might be 'enough' when it comes to your workouts, let's look at how you can progress with your chosen form of exercise.

To be able to progress in any form of exercise, we want to be using a technique called 'progressive overload'. When we exercise (for example when we go for a 5k run), we place stress on the body and this stress requires our bodies to make adaptations in order for us to recover from the exercise. Over time, as we adapt to the given stress, we learn to do that same exercise or stressor again but with less effort than before. Our body becomes able to complete the given demands and is therefore able to tolerate more. Progressive overload is the process of layering small increases in training, one on top of the other, session after session, across a period of time, so that you continue to improve at a given task. This could be applied to lots of styles of training, including weight training, running and swimming.

So, what happens within the body to allow this to occur? When we train, we place forces on our muscles, which is known as 'mechanical tension' and part of this involves inflicting a small amount of damage on our muscles. In response to more mechanical tension being placed upon the muscles, our bodies work to increase our ability to manage this level of mechanical tension again, as well as adapting to the tiny micro tears to our muscles that occur as part of this process. It's during this process that more blood flows to the muscles, which in turn improves nerve signalling, stores energy more efficiently and allows for the muscles to strengthen. These adaptations mean that with consistency and over time, when you try to complete the given demand again, for example running another 5k, your body will have become stronger in that given movement, which allows you to run faster, or for longer.

It's important to understand that this process can't be rushed. Increases in training have to be small so the body has a chance to adapt and recover. If we do too much, injury or fatigue can happen, but if each exercise is gradually progressed, enough food is consumed and adequate sleep is achieved, the body has a chance to adapt fully to make the exercise easier for you.

Key things to look out for

The most common ways that progressive overload can be applied – taking weight training as an example – is through intensity and volume, but there are also other ways to include it within your routine. Many people end up rushing the process and getting into situations where they can't progress, often because their ego has got in the way so working at the right tempo is important. These are the key areas to focus on with a view to building up progressive overload at a sensible pace:

- **Intensity** This means increasing the load every 1–4 weeks. A good way to do this is to start with a weight that feels comfortable but challenging for you, and then gradually increase it as the given rep range starts to feel easier.
- **Volume** This is the number of total reps performed for any given exercise. For example, if you did 3 sets of 10 reps at 10kg, your total volume load would be 300kg. If you were then to increase the reps to 3 x 11 the following week, your total volume load would be 330kg, meaning you'd placed greater stress on the body.
- **Tempo** This is the speed at which you do a rep. Many people I've trained have tended to rush through their reps without much thought, but manipulating tempos can be a really effective way to progressively overload an exercise. By slowing the tempo of an exercise, you increase the time in which the muscle in question is under tension, therefore making it work harder than if you had rushed the rep. An example could be slowing down the lowering or eccentric portion of your squat, pausing at

the bottom for a moment, before driving back up to standing.

- **Frequency** Increasing the amount of training you do per week can be a good way of progressively overloading the body, but it's essential to note that this isn't sensible for everyone. If you're a complete beginner starting with two days of training per week, it should be manageable to eventually increase this to three days a week, for example. However, regular or drastic increases can't be sustained over the long term and are not ideal for those who already train a lot each week. Remember that recovery is crucial to progression, and so having too much frequency can hinder rather than help your progress (I will explain more about this in the next chapter). A smart approach could be to spread your exercises over an additional training day. Let's say you train twice a week; you complete eight exercises per workout and you feel like you could be doing a little more. You could take those sixteen total exercises, add in two more, but spread them over three days. So now you are doing six exercises per workout, and eighteen total exercises per week. Adding a workout doesn't mean you have to make a huge jump in the total amount of work you complete. This is a great way of progressing while also ensuring you take adequate time to recover.

- **Improving form** For newbie lifters, simply working on improving the form of your exercises can be a way of challenging the body more each session. Spending a few weeks mastering form so you can move better is a method of gradual progression and a critical one for those new to lifting weights, for example. As the weights you are lifting go up, it's a skill to manage your whole body position under the increased load. Spending a few weeks really locking in your form is often essential in terms of achieving progress.

Above all, progressive overload should be gradual, regardless of which way you achieve it. It might not be sexy, but it's smart – and smart wins every time.

How do I start strength training?

When it comes to how you begin, it is worth saying that people often have a tendency to rush into exercise and lift as much as they can, or run as far as they can, as quickly as possible. Believe me when I say, slow and steady is the way to go. What we want is a gradual increase in activity. Ideally, that means doing a manageable amount, so we can recover adequately and it doesn't feel overbearing or like a chore. While this might seem counterintuitive to getting results, I learned the hard way that the 'more training the better' simply isn't the case.

If you've reached this point in the book and are thinking that perhaps strength training isn't for you, do please skip to page 227. If, however, you've decided it's something you are interested in and you are now wondering where to start on your strength training journey, please don't panic. This is by far the most common subject I am asked about online, and I can very much empathize with the daunting feeling of knowing you want to do something, but not having a clue how to begin!

Something reassuring to know is that apart from terrible form, which can be dangerous, there really is no wrong way to approach weight training. While, of course, it's not quite as simple as lacing up your trainers and setting out for a run, you're also very unlikely to fail when you decide to add some weights into your routine for the first time.

When it comes to starting your weight training journey, my number one piece of advice is to master the basics first. This means learning some key movement patterns using purely your own body weight before you start to add any load to the equation. These movements include:

1. Some form of squat, e.g. a goblet squat
2. Some form of hip hinge, e.g. a glute bridge

3. Some form of upper body pushing movement, both horizontal and vertical, e.g. a chest press and a military press
4. Some form of upper body pulling movement, both horizontal and vertical, e.g. a lateral pull-down and a three-point single arm row
5. Improving mobility, e.g. doing 90/90 rotations prior to your workout for hip mobility
6. Working on proprioception and stability, e.g. doing a single leg exercise within your routine
7. Core strength, e.g. doing some dead bugs within your routine
8. Locomotion, e.g. doing some walking lunges within your routine

When training clients on the gym floor, I'd usually spend time working on each of the above movements until the client felt confident, which is when you can add an additional load. Building this solid foundation will ensure that you prioritize form and quality of movement over just trying to wing it with weights.

So what might a training plan look like for someone who's never lifted weights?

I've listed some exercises below that I'd encourage you to try if you're unsure where to start with your weight training journey. These can help to build your confidence and set you off on a path of getting stronger. If you aren't familiar with these, you can find videos where I demonstrate them on my app: www.givemestrength.app.

Body weight squat or goblet squat

Start with your feet slightly wider than hip width apart and with your feet slightly turned out. From this position, bend at the knee, almost as if you're going to sit down on to a chair. Aim to lower down to a point where you have a 90-degree angle at the knee, while ensuring that your heels remain on the ground throughout the movement. From this position, drive up to your initial standing position and repeat.

Glute bridge from the floor

Lying on the floor, bend at the knee so the soles of your feet are flat to the floor and your feet are about hip width apart. From this position, drive the hips upwards, focusing on squeezing your glutes at the top before lowering slowly back down and repeating.

Glute bridge from a bench

Rest your upper back (your shoulder blades) on a box or bench that is roughly at knee height. With your feet planted on the floor about hip width apart, drive your hips up so you form a bridge position, before lowering back down and repeating. Make sure you focus on tucking the pelvis in a little at the top.

Shoulder taps

Come into a high plank position with your arms straight and your hands under your shoulders. Lift one hand and tap the opposite shoulder before placing it back down on the floor and repeating on the opposite side. The aim is to keep the pelvis still, so avoid rocking from side to side.

Plank hold

Place your elbows on to the floor, stacked underneath your shoulders, and then step your legs out so you create a straight line with your body. Aim to keep long through the back of the neck with your gaze down towards the floor. Squeeze the inner thighs together and hold for 20–30 seconds, or longer if you're able.

Walking lunge or static lunge

With your feet underneath your hips, take one step forwards and bend your knees so your back knee is just off the floor, then drive off from the back foot, step forwards with this foot and repeat the same motion. Keep going for 6–8 repetitions each side.

World's greatest stretch

From a high plank position (arms straight and hands under your shoulders), step one foot forwards so that it sits outside of the hand on the same side. Reach that hand upwards so you rotate through the upper body, then return it to the ground, step the leg back and repeat on the other side.

Standing swimmers

Imagine you're doing backstroke and then front stroke, but standing up.

The Pros and DOMS

While pushing yourself can bring many positives, such as a feeling of accomplishment, enjoying the progress you're making and improving form in the movements you're doing, I'm sure many of you know that feeling of waking up the day after a workout and struggling with muscle soreness. In fact, maybe this is why you haven't stuck with weight training in the long term?

This soreness is known as DOMS, which is short for Delayed Onset Muscle Soreness. This typically occurs around 24–72 hours post-workout, and normally happens when you utilize muscles you haven't worked before or exert yourself above and beyond what you usually do in a training session. Interestingly, we don't fully understand why there is a delay in the onset of soreness, which seems to occur during the later stages of the repair process.

Much of the soreness comes from the micro tears which are created in our tissue when we exercise. While the word tear can sound a little terrifying, they're nothing to worry about. Once these tears are created there is a need for us to repair them – and our magical bodies do that for us. But remember, we are not *aiming* for more soreness. It's important to be aware that there are two types of tissue repair that can occur:

- **Tissue remodelling** This is when you create so much damage that your body has to remodel the entire muscle fibre.
- **Tissue repair and strengthening** This is when there has been some localized damage but the tissue fibre itself is still functional, so the repair process actually increases the capacity of the tissue to tolerate the stimulus (i.e. to get stronger).

The first type of damage (tissue remodelling) is the one we want to try and avoid if possible. It can mean that you're so sore you can't train effectively. In this situation you're causing too much structural damage to the tissue, so it's impossible to recover efficiently and make progress. The second type of damage is the sweet spot; it's far less likely to create extreme soreness and allows you to gradually place more stimulus on the body, ultimately to get stronger.

It's essential to remember that soreness doesn't necessarily equal a 'good' workout. It might seem good to feel the results of your hard work, but consistently bombarding the body with too much stimulus can lead to fatigue, injury and – eventually – a loss of motivation.

It's difficult to avoid DOMS entirely though, and you might occasionally get it if you try a new exercise or push yourself beyond what you're used to. If this happens to you, it's a good idea to go for a gentle walk or swim or do something slower-paced to increase blood flow. You should also make sure you're eating a diet rich in protein, as well as getting good-quality sleep, as these will all aid your recovery.

What are workout splits and which is best for me?

You might have heard people who weight train talking about their 'workout splits'. This is a reference to how they've broken down and structured their workouts.

There are so many ways to write workout plans, and while I might sound like a stuck record at this point, there is no single best way to structure your training. Different splits suit different people, so I thought I'd share some of the most common types so you can work out which might best suit you and your training.

Full-body training split

This is a nice way to split your workout and helps to cover all the bases across a week of training. Personally, I tend to lean towards full-body workouts as every session is challenging and covers a range of different movements.

Full-body training is great for both beginners and

advanced lifters and can be really helpful in avoiding soreness in a particular muscle group. This is because the training is spread out across a few sessions rather than isolated to just one or two sessions per week.

With full-body training, we tend to (although not always) focus more on movements rather than particular muscle groups. These can be broken down into:

- Knee dominant movements (bilateral and unilateral). These involve an exercise where the knee joint is in flexion, for example a squat or a lunge.
- Hip dominant movements (bilateral and unilateral). These involve an exercise where the hips achieve flexion, for example a deadlift or a good morning.
- Upper push and pull, horizontal and vertical (bilateral and unilateral). These involve movements where you push (and then pull) a weight or object in a horizontal or vertical line, for example a lying dumbbell chest press or a lateral pull-down.
- Rotational movements. These involve movements where the trunk (torso) and/or body rotates, such as Russian twists or cable wood chops.
- Gait (walking, running, sprinting). This is how we move in locomotion, either through walking, running or sprinting.

While I'm keen not to oversimplify programming here, essentially you need to make sure you include each type of the above movements at the most basic level in your workout routine. That way your programme is far more likely to be balanced and effective. You can also find videos of these exercises on my app: www.givemestrength.app.

Upper/lower workouts

For those who don't enjoy full-body workouts, splitting the upper and lower body can be an effective way of breaking up your routine. I have used upper/lower splits many times in my own training, and I find it helpful if I'm looking to build lean muscle. The benefit of an upper/lower split is that, in theory, it allows for substantial rest and recovery during a week. For example, if you do legs on Monday and upper body on Tuesday, you might not train your legs again until Thursday, which allows them plenty of time to recover.

There are, however, some negatives to this training style. One is that it's not great for those who don't have lots of free time to train. If someone's schedule only allows them three workouts a week, an upper/lower split may not provide them with enough stimulus to elicit proper muscle growth.

Another situation where upper/lower splits may not be the best strategy is with advanced lifters, who want to hit high training volume and require more frequent and heavier training.

In summary, both training styles can be effective tools for gaining strength and seeing results. In many cases, splits often allow for more frequent training and better recovery. However, full-body workouts can provide a good training stimulus in a more time-efficient manner during the week. It depends on what your goals are, what your WHY is, what your schedule allows, what type of training you enjoy and what other exercise you might include in your current routine.

Split body part workouts

Although this isn't my favourite way to organize my workouts, some people really benefit from a split body part workout structure. This involves breaking the body down into muscle groups, for example, glutes and hamstrings, back and biceps, chest and triceps.

This style is typically synonymous with a bodybuilding style of training and allows time for an intense workout of a specific area of the body, with extra days for that area to recover before it is worked again. It's thought this helps target one or two muscle groups more specifically or intensively, with more sets and heavier reps.

While there are some pros to this type of training, it can be incredibly time-consuming and challenging to meet the schedule of training required to make sure each muscle group is covered at least once a week (but no more than twice a week). If one day's training is missed, it often means that a particular muscle group won't be worked until the following week, which can make progress more difficult to achieve. This style of training may work for those who have a lot of time to dedicate to being in the gym but for most people it is far more efficient to choose one of the other training styles instead.

8. When

Above all else, I hope it is clear by now that exercise must be something that you're able to stick to in the long term. That means that making it compatible with your lifestyle. Of course, having a routine for your workouts is important, but that counts for little if you can't implement consistency within your training. So, let's talk about how much training we should be doing, and how we can make a plan that really works for you.

How often should we move?

There is no optimum amount of exercise you can do each week because our training thresholds (the amount of exercise you can do each week) will vary substantially from person to person. For that reason, it is important to approach this question in an intuitive way and work out what is best for you. The first thing to consider is how many sessions you're able to consistently fit in each week. Our lives are so busy, and training can often get pushed lower and lower down the priority list. But it's important to create healthy habits with exercise and make sure you do carve out time for your training when you're able to.

Being realistic about this is key because it's not going to do wonders for your motivation when you plan to do five sessions and only manage two. So really think about what a genuinely realistic amount of training each week will be for you and try and build from there.

The next question is, of course, what is the desired outcome? Goals will dictate to a certain extent how much someone should be exercising each week. If you're planning to run a marathon in a few months' time, the chances are your miles per week are going to be ramping up and you'll feel an increasing demand on how much you are training. Similarly, if improving your overall physical strength is your goal, doing only one strength session a week might not be enough. So, try and work out how much might be needed to get you to your goal.

That said, if there is no specific goal you're working towards, a more abstract rule could be to roughly follow the current government guidelines, which suggest that we should be doing at least 150 minutes of exercise each week. You could break that down in whatever way works best for you.

Rest days – what, when, how, why?

As we discussed in the progressive overload section, any exercise we do is a stressor on the body, albeit (normally) a good one. But that stimulus requires us to adapt and recover in order to improve and get more efficient at dealing with the demands of exercise. Recovery is a complex topic; it's not just about taking a day off. There are many factors that play a part in our recovery – eating enough good-quality food and getting enough sleep are both essential, as are hydration and mobility. These make up the most important building blocks of a solid recovery routine and should be prioritized if you're training consistently. Your approach to rest days will also depend on what type of workout you're doing, your ability and both your training and biological ages too. Let's start with rest days.

Rest days are when you take a conscious break from doing a specific exercise. It doesn't have to mean that you lie in bed all day doing nothing, but you do give your body a break from any heavy demands. Activities such as gentle walking, swimming or cycling can be fine, but you're aiming to keep the amount of stress you place on the body during these days low, in order to feel recovered and rested.

As a general rule, you will likely need more days of rest if:

- In strength training, you lift heavy weights close to your max, and your workouts take about an hour.
- You are new to exercise or getting back into exercise after a break.
- You do impact forms of cardio, and you progress and push your limits by frequently hitting PBs with times or distance.
- You are overcoming illness or injury.

- You are pre/post-natal or returning to exercise after an extended break.

You likely need fewer rest days if:

- In strength training, you aren't pushing the loads you are lifting and are training at a comfortable level.
- You do a mixture of training where the intensities are spread. For example, doing a variety of higher and lower intensity training across your week with yoga, running, Pilates and hiking.
- You go for light jogs to get some fresh air and clear your head.
- You implement active recovery days by taking weeks off or training at a much lower intensity for a week to allow for recovery.

The most important take home is that you should listen to your body. As there is no one correct number of rest days that should be taken each week, it might be helpful instead to ask yourself the following questions:

- Do I feel energized and motivated in my training sessions?
- Do I feel energized when I wake up?
- Am I progressing in my workouts?
- Am I particularly sore regularly?
- Am I getting sick often?
- Am I getting injured often?

I hope these questions are helpful indicators as to whether you're doing enough or too much. Only you can really decide how much rest you need, depending on how much and what training you're doing, so play around with what works best for you and find your sustainable balance. Don't just choose an arbitrary number that may or may not be right.

A note on overtraining

As I shared in the first half of this book, I previously had a very rigid approach to my training. Sometimes I would get up at 4am to fit a gym session in before a busy day or cancel social plans because they didn't allow me to work out. I eventually realized that this attitude bred a very difficult relationship with exercise, where I couldn't allow myself even a single day off. What I learned from the experience is that any form of training, whether cycling, swimming or lifting weights in the gym, should be *flexible*. You need to be able to push yourself hard when you're feeling amazing, but also be kind to yourself and pull back when your body is telling you no. We're not robots! We have hormones, busy lives, families, friends and much more to contend with. A flexible approach to training is a winning formula.

A wise coach once told me that those who progress best in their training are the people who recognize that the recovery done outside of the gym is just as important as the work done in it. It's taken me a long time to realize the truth of that. 'Old Alice' didn't see the point of rest days. I would think: Why take a day off from the thing that makes me happy? In addition, rest days were also heavily associated with guilt, because I truly believed I couldn't stay small unless I maintained a high level of training every day. It's sad to think back to these times and remember how many crazily early alarms I set myself to squeeze in a workout, or how often I would head to the gym at 10pm, even though I was already exhausted.

Overtraining very often means that the body is under-recovering. It doesn't have adequate time and/or energy resources to properly recover from intense bouts of exercise, which can lead to the body having to work much harder to recover. If the training threshold remains too high (we will all have different thresholds at which we can operate, so there is no specific definition of how much training is too much), at some point our bodies will start to show signs they're struggling. This could involve (but isn't exclusive to) persistent fatigue, repetitive injuries that don't seem to improve, sleep disruption, mood swings, brain fog and a general lack of motivation.

We know exercise is important – it's even a personal passion of mine – but it's vital to understand that we can have too much of a good thing. Sadly, exercise can be harmfully addictive and while it might seem like a good idea to spend two hours in the gym regularly, in the hope it will help you to reach your goal quicker, the reality is that without adequate recovery between sessions, progress simply won't be sustainable in the long term, even if you see results in the short term. I want to help you understand why rest is important, and how you can use it to your advantage to get more from your exercise.

Optimizing recovery

There are other ways in which you can help your body to recover from training, in addition to rest days. Below I've included six things you can do to really help optimize the process and make sure you feel your best.

Sleep

Sleep is our hidden superpower. It's something we should all be prioritizing as an important element of our health and wellbeing, and yet we so often overlook or forget about it when it comes to feeling our best.

In very basic terms, there are two different types of sleep: REM and NREM. REM stands for 'rapid eye movement' and it's during these phases of sleep that our dreams occur. NREM is 'non-rapid eye movement' sleep and occurs in three stages. It's during the deeper phase three of NREM sleep that the magic happens; this is when our bodies repair our muscles, strengthen our immune systems, manage our hormones and sort our memories. We all know how a poor night's sleep or a consecutive run of poor sleep can make us feel. It can impact every aspect of our wellbeing.

It's understandable that sleep can't always be our number one priority but at aiming for 7–9 hours of sleep each night as often as possible is going to really help your recovery and fitness. If you are nowhere near 7–9 hours currently, it's still worth trying to move closer to that target. If you can get an extra 20–30 minutes' sleep by altering some daily habits, it's definitely worth it. The benefits of good sleep and recovery accumulate over time.

Nutrition

Eating enough to help your body recover well from training is also hugely important. The food we eat ensures that our body has enough energy to recover from the demands we place upon it and eating a good balance of protein, fats and carbohydrates is essential. I'm not a nutritionist so I won't go into too much depth here, but from a personal perspective, I used to be that girl who feared carbs, as many people do. Ultimately, cutting out a whole food group had a really negative impact on my energy. Of course, I 'pushed through', thinking I simply wasn't disciplined enough. But the reality was that my body didn't have enough fuel to handle the demands I was placing upon it. The single biggest difference that I have made to my training, beyond doing less, has been starting to eat enough carbs. And by enough, I mean carbohydrates at every meal, whether it's sweet potato, oats or rice. I've had to learn that carbohydrates are not the devil, and they're not going to make you gain weight overnight, or even in the long term.

Without being too specific, my advice is to use the 'trial and error' method with your diet. Add some carbs around your training to start with, some before and some after, and see if it helps with how you feel. Protein is also important, and especially so if you're exercising. Having a protein source, whether it's tofu, fish, chicken or eggs at *every* meal will help with hitting a daily protein target without needing to macro count every gram.

And finally, don't forget your fats. Whether it's Greek yogurt, avocado or nuts, including these regularly across your week will certainly help you to keep feeling at your best.

Movement

No, I don't mean doing a workout to recover from a workout! I mean some very slow, very gentle movement to encourage blood flow and aid the recovery process. On my rest days, I often focus on mobility to aid my recovery. This generally includes a full-body stretch and a wiggle, which helps to minimize areas of tightness and increase blood flow round the body and improves flexibility both during and outside of your training.

Aside from working on mobility, I'm not going to say don't do anything at all on your rest days. A gentle walk, cycle or anything that's very low intensity can be a good way of still getting the mental health benefits of movement without doing anything that's going to be too taxing on the body. But do please be aware, more steps = more energy output, which can tip the scales in terms of positive and negative outcomes. While some movement can be great, be mindful that slowing down and doing very little might also be just what your body needs. Be intuitive with this. If you wake up on your rest day with oodles of energy, by all means go for a walk. But if your body is saying, 'I need to slow down a little', listen to those signals and take your foot off the gas for a day. I promise that this will help your training and progress, not hinder it.

Hydration

This might sound like an obvious one, but it's worth stressing. Hydration is a crucial part of recovery and general wellbeing. We've probably all been told we need to drink a bit more water, but do you actually know why?

Water makes up 75 per cent of both our blood and our muscles. It's such a huge component of our physical make-up, so even the slightest drop in hydration levels can cause you to feel a bit off. When it comes to remembering to drink enough, the best thing you can do is buy a water bottle to carry around with you. I know it sounds like very generic advice, but it's really the only way to ensure that you are actively being reminded to drink a little more throughout the day.

Another thing to try if you're someone who exercises

and sweats a lot is to use rehydration (electrolyte) tablets. They're something I personally find useful if I'm having a week where I exercise regularly, and I find they can make me feel a lot better post-workout compared to just drinking some water.

Non-sleep deep rest (NSDR)

This is something I'm incorporating a lot more into my balanced life since recovering from my disordered approach to diet and exercise. Many of us live our lives at a relatively fast pace, whether it's running from one work commitment to the next or chasing after a small child. Life can be stressful and sometimes overwhelming, which isn't conducive to efficient recovery from training. While such day-to-day stresses are often unavoidable, we *can* learn to manually turn our 'stress dial' down, so that we ease the pressure on ourselves.

We all have two states within our autonomic nervous system: sympathetic (fight or flight) and parasympathetic (rest and digest). Unlike our caveman ancestors, we are unlikely to need to fight for our food or run away from predators, but an example of a time when you might find yourself in a sympathetic state would be before an important meeting or exam. Your heart races a little quicker, you might produce more saliva and your muscles might contract. These are all signs that you're in a fight or flight state. While this is often normal and necessary, what isn't normal is to spend too much time in this stressed state. Learning to turn the dial down and to return to a rest and digest state can be a really helpful tool in managing the body's overall stress levels.

One way to achieve this is with non-sleep deep rest. NSDR isn't intended to induce sleep, but instead involves a dreamy, semi-focused state that often occurs just before you fall asleep. You're still awake, but your awareness of space and time isn't totally under your conscious control.

One way you can achieve this is by practicing yoga nidra. It may sound a bit woo-woo, but bear with me. Yoga nidra is a very slow form of yoga where you lie down and listen to a structured meditation that guides you through the five layers of self. Each layer fades as you move from one to the next, leaving you in a state of deep rest.

You can find free examples of these kinds of meditation online. As a chronic 'doer' I find it really helps me to slow down and switch my stressed and overwhelmed state to one that is much calmer and has more clarity.

Breathwork

Another way to pull back from that stressed state is with breathwork. It's one of my favourite things in my 'chill out' toolkit and I use it on almost a daily basis. When you need to reassess your whole approach to health and wellbeing, you realize that it's often the things you dismiss as 'fluffy' that can have the biggest impact. I'm a naturally anxious person and I always have been, so my tendency is to find myself in a default stressed state. This means I really need to be conscious of learning coping strategies to help counteract my anxiety, so I can recover from the stress I put on my body, which in turn means I don't find myself burning out after a few weeks or months of intense work.

Simply slowing our breath down and making a conscious effort to breathe a little deeper and to really focus on the slow inhale and exhale of our breath can help to bring us back from a state of stress to a state of rest and digest. My favourite way to do this is with something called square breathing. It might take a little while for you to get used to doing it, but it's such a great technique to use at any point, anywhere you might need it. Here's how to do it:

Breathe in for four counts, hold for four counts, exhale for four counts and then hold again for four counts. Repeat this for a few minutes, or as long as you need until you feel yourself calming down.

If you do this slowly and in a controlled way, preferably in a comfortable seated position or lying down, it can really help you to find a calmer state of being. This, in turn, can help you to minimize the stress you experience in other areas of your life.

Rest day guilt

Rest day guilt is something that I certainly experienced back in my overtraining days, and I want to help you avoid it. Overcoming this guilt is challenging, but it's what you need to really get the most from your workouts, and to have a healthy long-term relationship with exercise.

I'll give you the reminder that I give all my clients: if training for life is the goal, then you're in no rush. It will always be there. It will always be something you can pick up and put back down as many times as you want. What won't always be there is your health if you continue to override the need for breaks from working out. Understanding that more doesn't equal better when it comes to exercise is so essential; it can be the difference between feeling okay and feeling your very best.

It's fine to feel a little lazy, or to have a day where you don't want to move at all. In fact, indulge in it and enjoy it, because it means that the next time you work out you're going to have so much energy to throw at it and will get more from your session as a result. So please don't feel guilty for simply doing what your body genuinely needs. You're not lazy or unmotivated or lacking in discipline; you're a human, not a robot.

When overtraining goes wrong

I spoke in Part 1 about losing my menstrual cycle. This symptom is something that many more women are now openly speaking about, as well as something medical practitioners are being made more aware of. However, when it happened to me there was very little information available on the subject. My issue was totally due to overtraining, and it's a scary example of what can happen if adequate rest isn't factored in.

What I now know was that I was suffering from 'hypothalamic amenorrhea'; a condition that causes your period to stop and can lead to further health problems if left untreated. As I described earlier, I personally only found this out through the great fortune of meeting Emma Cannon.

Hypothalamic amenorrhea can be caused by a number of factors, including stress, low energy availability, a low body fat percentage and doing too much exercise. I know for certain that mine was a combination of not eating enough and doing too much exercise. I'm often asked why I didn't worry or seek advice after going so long without a period, but I was on the contraceptive pill for a large period of my experience of amenorrhea, which masked the reality of my cycle. I then assumed that I hadn't got my period back because I had recently come off the pill. It was only after a substantial period of time that I sought help, and I'm sure many other women find themselves in a similar position.

I know from personal experience how easy it is to overtrain, and it's something a lot of people fall victim to. When you love to exercise and it becomes your coping mechanism and an escape from many of life's stressors, throwing yourself into more movement can even seem like a sensible thing to do. The reality is that when we continuously override our need to rest and recover, our bodies have to adjust by down-regulating vital functions, such as our menstrual cycle, to preserve energy for our most basic bodily functions.

Hypothalamic amenorrhea is something that we now describe under the umbrella term of RED-S, or Relative Energy Deficiency in Sport. The official definition of RED-S is impaired physiological functioning caused by relative energy deficiency. It includes, but is not limited to, impairments of metabolic rate, menstrual function, bone health, immunity, protein synthesis and cardiovascular health.

I think one difficult thing to untangle is realizing when your routine has tipped into being problematic. I was convinced for a very long time that I didn't have a problem because I still ate every day and had one lower intensity workout a week.

You don't have to be feeling or looking your smallest to suffer with RED-S. For example, an acute bout of stress or trauma can disrupt your cycle without your body weight changing at all. But in a sport and exercise context, it most commonly occurs when low energy availability is paired with a lack of adequate recovery. While the following list certainly isn't exhaustive, symptoms can include changes to the menstrual cycle, drops in performance, weight loss, mood changes, heart problems, loss of cognitive functions (for example difficulty focusing), increased injury, sleep pattern disruption, fatigue and increased illness.

Sufferers don't necessarily experience all these symptoms. I certainly didn't encounter every one of them, but it's important to know that the condition can present itself in different ways. It's also important to remember that it can impact people of all shapes and sizes, in any background or sport. It's not just about being incredibly thin. It's about how much stress you put on your body at a given time, that may cause it to halt certain processes for self-preservation.

If you ever find yourself experiencing menstrual disruption, my best advice would be to speak to a medical professional. Periods can go MIA for various reasons, and many of the above symptoms could be other health-related issues.

Having gone through the experience myself, I feel very passionate about speaking to women about the dangers of doing too much. My missing period was the catalyst for the major life change that I embarked on, and I'm so proud to now be in a place where I have regained a regular cycle. The fine balance between doing enough and too much can be tricky to get right, and if you're struggling to know how much counts as excessive, it's sometimes far better to have someone to help you to figure that out rather than constantly overriding any doubts you might have.

Here is a useful series of questions to help you decide whether you're sufficiently rested and ready to exercise at any given time. I've used this with many of my clients before and it serves as a tangible way of checking in with yourself and pausing and reflecting, rather than simply pushing yourself to work out, which might not be what your body needs. Before each session, I want you to ask yourself the following simple questions:

1. Do I feel energized and motivated for today's workout?
2. Does my body feel rested and ready for today's workout?
3. Have I eaten enough to fuel today's workout?
4. Have I had enough sleep to do today's workout?
5. What would happen if I didn't exercise today?

It's important to be honest when answering these questions. It will help you to be more intuitive with how you're really feeling, and in turn allow you to rest more intuitively too. Being flexible will allow you to recognize that you *can* take another rest day if you need one, which in turn may well mean that you'll be able to have a full training schedule the following week, as by then you'll be feeling sufficiently rested and recovered.

The final question in the list above is key, and I sometimes put it to myself twice, just to be sure. We often catastrophize about what might happen if we skip a single workout, when the reality is that nothing will happen. If anything, taking a pause could well be an important building block for a more intuitive and long-lasting relationship with exercise.

Missing a gym session or two (or even three) will

have no impact on your body or your progress. We aren't a product of what we do once. Just as you don't get instantly stronger in a single gym session, you also don't lose all your progress by missing one. If every week you are skipping multiple gym sessions, of course that will have an impact. But simply missing a few here and there, which is completely normal, is not going to make any difference.

Putting all the pieces together

In these chapters, I've shown you everything I had to do to relearn and heal my relationship with exercise. I know it isn't realistic to try and eliminate the diet culture hangovers of working out to punish ourselves and to burn calories, and constantly centring everything around losing weight. This is because we're existing in an environment that is determined to feed us a very binary narrative of exercise. But being able to consciously challenge this outdated and unsustainable way of approaching exercise can change everything. So how do you put all these pieces of information together to form your new way of moving and enjoying exercise? The first thing I'd encourage you to do is to wipe the slate clean. Forget all that's gone before, and simply focus on your new 'after'.

Here are the key learnings to take from these sections. If nothing else, I hope these resonate with you and can go some way to improving your relationship with exercise:

1. Ditch – or slowly wean yourself off – the scales. These are not going to be reflective of your training progress, so stop punishing yourself by stepping on them and expecting them to make you feel good.
2. Work out your macro goal (your WHY), which will help you to create a plan that actually gets you where you want to be rather than chasing other people's version of success.
3. Find a way of moving your body that you genuinely enjoy rather than because it burns the most calories.
4. Start tracking your progress in tangible metrics.
5. Work on managing your EAT energy exposure by being more mindful of how you increase your NEAT energy – make small changes to your daily routine without going crazy or overdoing it.
6. Be genuinely content with your routine. It has to work for you, and that's crucial.
7. Know that – very often – less is more.
8. Remember that this journey won't be linear. Roll with the punches and try and overcome the days where you feel like you're taking steps backwards. I promise you aren't.

9. Beyond your body

So far, I've spoken a lot about the specifics of exercise. Finding your WHY, working out your WHAT and then thinking about your HOW and your WHEN will all help you to carve out a fresh and healthy approach to exercise. However, we know that health isn't just about exercising in the right way and eating a nutritious and balanced diet. Our overall wellbeing is complex and there are so many elements that need to be considered beyond what we put into and how we move our bodies if we truly want to be happy, healthy beings.

I wanted to share in this final section some of the things outside of the gym that have really helped me to feel my best, all of which have nothing to do with the way I look. My hope is that once you've set a plan in place for your relationship with exercise, you can also look to this section for ways to enhance that part of your life with self-care.

I have done a lot of reading and researching around the things we can do that are grounded in science and that directly benefit our physical and/or mental health. Below I've written about five things I now do regularly that have helped me to manage stress and anxiety, sleep better and, ultimately, live a happier and more fulfilled life.

Journalling

I started keeping a journal when I began therapy a few years ago. My therapist suggested it as a way to brain-dump the stuff I'd been feeling in one place. I scoffed at the idea at first, but then decided to give it a go.

Fast-forward to now and journalling is part of my daily routine. It's not that it changes anything huge in the moment, but it does help me to offload the stresses and worries of each day, which means I sleep more easily and don't feel my emotions snowballing as they have done in the past.

That first time, I started with a blank page and felt myself staring down at it, unsure what to write. Initially I simply wrote down what I had done each day. Then, slowly but surely, I got comfortable with relaying what I was feeling with absolute honesty – the good, the bad and the ugly, with zero judgement. You see, the benefit of a journal is that it's a completely passive listener, so the stuff you bury deep down and the things you hold back from saying for fear of judgement can all be shared with 100 per cent privacy.

When you're on a journey towards finding your balance and unlearning the things that have been weighing you down, it can be helpful to express in writing how you're feeling about it all. If you had a day when you were inclined to restrict, write it down. If you have a day when you binge-ate, write it down. It can be incredibly powerful to release your thoughts on to the page. I promise you, journalling will make a difference to how you feel.

Being in nature

I'm not saying that you should immediately head outdoors and start hugging trees but hear me out. Being in nature is *really* good for us. It has been found to help with mental health problems such as anxiety and depression, but even if you're not struggling with these conditions, the great outdoors has been shown to reduce stress and increase a sense of calm that can be hard to achieve anywhere else.

A while ago, I started making it a personal priority to spend time in nature whenever possible during my week, and as a non-negotiable on my weekends. Every time I got outdoors (and put my phone away) I felt *so* much better. This may in part be due to the impact that natural light can have on us. Our eyes are directly connected to our brains and exposure to natural light, particularly early in the day, can really anchor us to our circadian rhythm and ensure that we are feeling awake and then sleepy at the right points during our wake–sleep cycle. It's the reason why if I am going to get outside, I try and do it in the early part of the day.

One way to achieve this could be to use one of your lower-intensity movement days to find some green space and spend time in nature, whether going for a bike ride or even just walking around. Okay, it might feel a little bit silly at first, but you're doing two things – walking and noticing the beauty of nature – that are scientifically proven to improve your physical and mental health. If you spend a lot of time in front of a screen, or live in a big city, this is even more of a reason to prioritize spending time in nature whenever possible.

Meditating

I'm sure it's no surprise to you that I've featured meditation here. It's become such a buzzword in the wellness world, but I do genuinely believe that it can have a powerful impact on how we feel.

You might be surprised to hear that despite my total belief that meditation is good for me, I'm also pretty awful at it. I tried the traditional meditation methods. I downloaded the apps and worked really hard to try and bring myself to a state of calm. But no matter how hard I tried, I always ended up a little bored, fidgety and frustrated. I felt like I must be doing something wrong rather than it just not being right for me.

I started to read more about what meditation really was. The more I understood that it was simply the practice of focusing on the mind or on a particular object, or training our attention and awareness to achieve a mentally clear and emotionally calm and stable state, the more I realized I might be able to achieve those same goals in other ways.

So, my ways of meditating don't include sitting in a cross-legged position or lying down with my eyes closed. Instead, I concentrate on doing something but bringing my absolute focus and attention to that practice. I often find that cooking, walking or ironing allow me to find this state most easily. (I know, ironing!)

The benefits can be far-reaching. Meditation allows us to turn that stress dial down, so I want to encourage you not to write it off if you struggle with it initially like I once did. Instead, reframe and refocus what meditation might look like to you. Whatever it may be, the practice is in training your mind, focusing on that activity alone. Try to quieten the other noise (although it may still creep in sometimes) and have a clear intention of allowing your brain to switch off.

Relationships

Social connection is so essential to our wellbeing, and yet very often, it gets neglected. Human beings are social creatures and while the extent of our sociability will vary from person to person, we all thrive on interaction with others.

Stats show that loneliness is on the rise in the UK,

with many of us finding ourselves communicating through and using screens to such an extent that we can go a whole day, if not longer, without speaking to another human being.

Some of this is unavoidable and I understand that. But prioritizing social connection can take you out of a place where your world revolves around food and exercise, and instead allows you to enjoy life and create connections with friends that can help to keep you in a balanced and healthy place. I told myself that I was a 'home person' and an 'introvert' for so long, but the reality was that I was scared of socializing because it meant navigating unknown situations involving food, and the risk of feeling out of control. It genuinely feels difficult to admit this, but it's the truth. I cancelled so many plans that revolved around food, or conveniently showed up to events having already eaten because the fear of the unknown was too much for me to manage. I always had an excuse. Cancelling was the easiest option as it meant no questions, and so my social interactions dwindled at the point when I probably needed them the most.

I've spent the last few years rebuilding many of the relationships that were damaged through my eating disorder. I feel so incredibly lucky that Paddy stuck by me, as did many of my close friends, but I'd be lying if I said that some of my relationships weren't affected by it. Overcoming my fears of being out of control, eating out and socializing had to be worked on. I challenged myself to say 'yes' to more, and I do now go out of my comfort zone when it comes to where I eat and what I order. It wasn't easy, but the reward of being able to have genuine fun with my friends again has been so unbelievably worth it.

I want you to realize that human connection and truly living your life arguably *is* your health and wellbeing. In all honesty, the hours spent in the gym or the healthy meals you whip up won't make you happy if you don't have some real fun and enjoyment thrown in there too. I spent too long sacrificing those things in the pursuit of wellness, only to realize that my whole approach was (ironically) profoundly bad for my health. Those weekends where you have a drunken takeaway after a night out, a glass of wine with the girls or a pizza night with the kids? They're important too. Please don't forget that.

A final note from me

And so we reach the end of this book. Writing *Give Me Strength* has been by far the most cathartic project I've ever worked on, and it's something I have thrown my heart and soul into. I've bared all and been brutally honest and I hope that has resonated with you. I wanted to tell you my real story, from start to finish, and I'm incredibly grateful to you for reading it.

I spent so many years hating my body, punishing myself and trying to be as slim as I could, because I thought that was what would make me happy. I thought that if I changed my body, I'd finally be more desirable, more inspirational and more acceptable. How wrong I was. I'm done with that damaging narrative. Now, I want to be the change I want to see in the world myself. I want young girls to read this book and totally avoid the toxic path that I and so many others fell into. I want to see a major shake-up in the fitness industry, where it ditches the harmful techniques that are far too often used to shame people into exercising. I want everyone to find a joyful way of moving their bodies that isn't rooted in simply making themselves smaller. And I want the world to wake up to how damaging it is to tell us that in doing so, we will be happier.

Ultimately, I want you to find peace and happiness within yourself and your body.

Give Me Strength is a tour of my chaotic journey, told with unflinching honesty. Thankfully this story has a happy ending. Although it was a challenging process, I've turned my back on everything that made me miserable and chosen genuine health and joy instead. I hope that in reading this book, you're now ready to start day one of your own journey. Please do keep me posted with how you get on.

All my love,
Alice x

Acknowledgements

Without it sounding too much of a cliché, this book has been such a labour of love. Over the course of a year, I poured everything I could into making this book as real, truthful and useful as I possibly could, sharing the bare reality of what has been a rollercoaster ten years lived online. It has been such a journey, and I am forever grateful to every single person who has picked it up and read it. It hasn't been easy to bare all, but it's been the most freeing journey to go on.

There are so many people to thank for making this book what it is.

The first person is my editor, Amy. When we first came together and had initial conversations about writing a book, Amy had complete trust in me when I shared my vision. I'd wanted to write this book for a long time but it was Amy who took a chance on me and believed in the importance of sharing the journey I'd been on since my last book. Where other editors might have tried to shoehorn the book into a specific formula just to sell copies, Amy placed total faith in my vision to look back and reflect on all that I've learned over my career, with the aim of offering solidarity and a clearer way forward for other women.

The next person to thank is my manager, Issy. Writing

this book, as well as almost everything I've ever done in my career, wouldn't have been possible without Issy. When I think back to when we first met, there was something about Issy that I was drawn to. She is no-nonsense, incredibly hard-working, passionate, driven and always thinking outside of the box. Every single part of what I do is thanks to her and her total belief in me. I honestly couldn't do any of it without her.

Paddy and my family also deserve a mention, of course. They have undoubtedly influenced this book, and me, and supported the journey of me writing it. From many tears shed during the writing process, to the endless hours of writing and re-writing, they have been there as my number one cheerleaders, lifting me up when I needed it and celebrating every win, no matter how small. I can be the happy person I am today because of them, and I am eternally grateful for their love and support.

The wider team at Penguin deserve a huge thank you too. There is SO much work that goes into creating a book, and the publishing team work tirelessly to make sure that everything is the best it can possibly be. From copy-editing and proofreading my words, to designing the cover, to the marketing, publicity and sales strategy, the following people are crucial cogs in the machine of creating this book. They are: Claire Collins, Corinna Bolino, Annie Moore, Natalie Wall, Sara Granger and Emma Pidsley. Thank you so much.

My final thanks go to you. This book was written for

the women who see themselves in my journey. I hope I've helped you to see that there is another way to health and happiness, and I wish you all the love on your own journey.

Alice x